Unlearning Stress

Creating an Easier, Healthier, More Balanced Life

For easier days

Jim Rohr

James Rohr, L.Ac.

Coyote Road Press

This book is not intended as a substitute for the medical advice of physicians. The reader should regularly consult a physician in matters relating to his/her health and particularly with respect to any symptoms that may require diagnosis or medical attention.

Printed in the United States of America.

First Printing, 2013

ISBN 978-0-9898614-1-0

Coyote Road Press

1410 20th St Suite 218

Miami Beach, FL 33139

www.coyoteroadpress.com

Illustrations by: Kevin Coffey

Cover design by: Diana Perez

To all of my patients, especially those in the very beginning of my practice, who were willing to let some kid just out of school be their doctor. And to all the patients who have blessed me with the opportunity to work on them since those first days, thank you for all you have taught and shared with me.

Advanced praise for Unlearning Stress

"This is the book to read if you want to have a different, more sublime experience of life. These 10 practices, clearly and beautifully stated, are what ancient sages taught and modern science is con firming. Sit down and read this book. Then put it into practice. I have every confidence you will see the changes." Karen Koffler, MD, Medical Director of Canyon Ranch Hotel & Spa Miami Beach.

"James is a master healer with a brilliant mind, a big heart, and a deep soul. His new book *Unlearning Stress* is a testament to his gifts. This is much more than a book, but a companion for health, healing and the creation of a vibrant life. This is not your typical self-help or wellness book; you will find clear guidance and practical wisdom for every day of your life. You are guaranteed to learn something new and vital to your health along the way. This is an important contribution to any home library or path to health and well-being." —Jonathan Ellerby, Ph.D. CEO *TAO Inspired Living,* author of *Inspiration Deficit Disorder.*

"*Unlearning Stress* gives you the tools to thrive—mind, body, and spirit. I can't wait to get this book in the hands of my patients." —Leslie Mendoza Temple, MD, Clinical Assistant Professor, Family Medicine, University of Chicago Pritzker School of Medicine, Medical Director, Integrative Medicine Program NorthShore University HealthSystem

"*Unlearning Stress* is a practical and easy to read guide that bring you the latest techniques to combat the high intensity demands of the modern lifestyle." — Eva Ritvo, MD Co-author of *The Beauty Prescription* and *The Concise Guide to Marriage and Family Therapy.*

"*Unlearning Stress* takes readers thru a process to become better versions of themselves. The steps James discusses are time-tested, vital components for a balanced and healthy life." —Brad Kerschensteiner, LMFT, founder of the Integrative Change Network

"In my practice I look for any tools or resources that will help my athletes and patients gain an edge with their healing. James' book is a welcome addition to help decrease stress so they can get back to enjoying their lives to the fullest." —Chris Herrera, DPT CSCS USAW

Acknowledgments

Many people, directly and indirectly, helped to bring this book into fruition: Dr. Karen Koffler for all the opportunities she has given me over the years, Gwen Hurd for her tireless patience with all the various drafts, Lesley Scott who helped to give shape, vision, and enthusiasm to this project, all of my teachers and mentors across various disciplines, acupuncture colleagues and associates, and of course, my loving family. Thank you all.

Any errors are all mine and should in no way be held against any of these wonderful people who took the time to care about something and someone other than themselves.

Table of Content

Introduction

Can you imagine a world where instead of asking about your symptoms, your doctor asks if you are fulfilling your life's mission? What if 'how is your chronic illness?' is replaced with 'how can I help you fulfill your destiny?'

What if I were to suggest that 'health' has absolutely nothing to do with the presence or absence of symptoms?

And what if I suggested that an optimal life is one that is lived in harmony between your body's constitution and your natural environment?

I have treated billionaires and movie stars, top level athletes and high powered CEO's. I have also treated cancer patients, terminal patients, weekend warriors, pregnant moms, annoyed teenagers, stressed out singles, and more. What they have taught me is that no matter how much money, power, or celebrity you have, the quality of life, true Health of the highest order, has much more to do with how well you know yourself and can follow your inner direction than anything to do with your symptoms. Symptoms, and the stress they cause, may come and go, they may stay for a long time, but what are you doing with your life in the meantime?

Stress is a parasite. It will eat and devour everything good inside of you until all that remains is sickness. Lethargy, inflammation, terrible relationships, addictions, and much much more become the norm. The manifestations of stress are many. But you already know this, which is why you're flipping thru a book about overcoming stress.

The good news is that most of the stress most of us are facing is learned. And if it is learned, then you can unlearn it. We are taught, consciously or unconsciously, to care about things that are big-picture insignificant. We are allowing our perceptions and expectations to drive the bus, and we are helpless passengers, hoping to get to our destination. So, if the bus careens out of control, we're going with it. The time has come to take back the driver's seat and grab the wheel.

Picture a young and healthy sprout for a watermelon. Given the right environment and tender loving care, this seedling will grow to provide a delicious treat for someone.

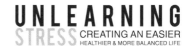

Now, take this seedling and throw it in a patch of winter snow. A delicious watermelon doesn't seem so likely anymore.

Picture yourself going from doctor to acupuncturist to chiropractor to massage therapist, pharmaceutical to nutraceutical, yoga class to Pilates, self-help book to online health blogs, all in an attempt to feel better. Maybe you're searching for treatments to your chronic fatigue, pain, inflammation, anxiety, etc. Now imagine you're doing that while being totally stressed out, eating fast food, checking your email 80,000 times a day, arguing with your spouse, getting agitated about work deadlines, and feeling underappreciated. While your treatment regimen may be good, your other lifestyle choices are the equivalent of pouring cement (or a patch of snow) on our happy little seedlings. A healthy version of you doesn't seem so likely anymore.

Unlearning Stress provides you with a bunch of tools to nurture the seed of wellness inside of all of us. The suggestions within will assist you in feeling more free, inspired, and healthier. Do you deserve an easier life? I think so. Perhaps you have never been taught how to live an easier life. This book will give you the tools you need to begin to rewrite your story, to unlearn what has gotten you so out of whack. Whether you are navigating the darkness of a scary prognosis or simply want to overcome the malaise of your day to day routine, *Unlearning Stress* is for you.

Getting to a healthier, happier version of you demands awareness about who you are and the environment you continue to be in. The 'environment' can be the weather, the physical space around us, what we eat and drink, our home and work lives and those we spend time with, among others.

Finding balance between your internal world and your outer is something the Taoists were teaching thousands of years ago. Whether we like it or not, everything is connected. Compartmentalization doesn't exist. We cannot spend 14 hours a day at a job that we hate and think that it doesn't have an effect on our health.

You are now invited to step off of the merry go round of living according to how people think you should be living. Begin to free yourself from the confines of stress. This book is here to give you techniques to begin to discover you, your true being, for a more inspired and free internal life, day after day, season after season, year after year.

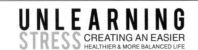

WHAT IS 'UNLEARNING'?

Unlearning is the deleting of files that no longer work for you. This is examining who you are and what are your motivations, habits, and decisions. What choices do you make day after day, month and year after year? What choices do you make thousands of times a day, moments after moments, about how you feel or what you expect yourself to be doing/accomplishing/behaving?

I start from the premise that you are enough without any cultural programming. No one needed to tell you how to behave in order to make you a better, more complete human being. We cannot improve upon a masterpiece. And yet, the modern lifestyle is attempting to do just that. We are forgetting our underlying nature, or natural state of 'being'. We are consumed with 'doing', chasing after some invisible reward of praise or meeting expectations.

In *Unlearning Stress,* you will be shown different ways of 'being' to help you unlearn those acquired suggestions of how you should behave, or what you should care about, or what you need to be accomplishing. I give you the tools to identify and delete those toxic files and return you to the present moment. Perhaps you'll meet yourself for the first time in a long time.

ABOUT UNLEARNING STRESS

The time has come to wake up. We'll do that thru cultivating awareness, learning about who we are, experimenting with various types of being, and focusing on what we want from this trip around the sun. The more you know about yourself, and the more you pay attention to your mental, social, and physical environment, the more likely you will be able to create the balance and freedom you want.

#1 Be Present. Aka Breathing 101. Just because you breathe enough to remain alive doesn't mean you've experienced the true power of deep abdominal breaths of the highest quality. This critical tool is free and always available. *Be Present* teaches the basics of breath to help you attain a higher level of awareness, enjoy a more open heart and quiet the mind.

#2 Be Calm. Calm is pretty much the opposite of what's going on with most of us. There is a struggle between the two major nervous systems in the body.

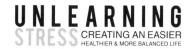

While the "Ah, nice, resting and relaxing" system wants to prevail, it's generally being muscled out of the way and run roughshod by the system concerned with "uh oh, should I fight? Should I flee?" Learning to gently disengage from one and tap into the other is the key to enduring long periods of stress and to ultimately liberating yourself from the entire stress cycle.

#3 Be Seated. Stress can be like a wet blanket over our fire of desire and passion. *Be Seated* is the antidote to that feeling of light and warmth fading within. To activate this resilience, I offer a variety of mindfulness options. Meditating doesn't require a big fuss, extensive rituals or even special rooms. There are plenty of options to choose from, even for the most ornery of restless, stressed-out, anti-meditators.

#4 Be Nourished. You are what eat. And what you eat, contributes mightily to how much your body and mind perceive stress. An inflamed body leads to an inflamed emotional mind. *Be Nourished* is chock-full of reasons why food really is medicine. If you put chocolate pudding into your car's gas tank, would you expect it to run very well? Learn how to fuel up properly to put yourself in the position to relax and chill out.

#5 Be Grateful. Not sure what to be grateful for? In this chapter, you will see that gratitude is the secret "Open, Sesame!" command to all kinds of freedom. You may even plant the seeds of gratitude in the most unlikely places. A well-placed 'thank you' can completely defuse a volatile situation. What if you could unlearn all the reasons you were stressed out and arrive at a heartfelt and meaningful 'thank you' to all those things that have you stressed out in the first place?

#6 Be Connected. Being connected is a critical component to healthy aging. Connect with your laugh. Connect with your pets. And connect with some romantic partners. There are also some 'advanced' lessons from those wise ancient Taoists to add some zest to your life. These will take you from stressed to sublime!

#7 Be Active. Movement is one of the time-honored secrets to breaking physical and emotional stagnation. To help you get your frolic on, I have suggestions from top movement experts along with the energy of Traditional Chinese Medicine and the wisdom of Qi. Many people use exercise to help

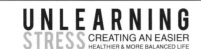

cope with stress, but this look at movement takes you to a deeper level, where movement across all levels of the mind/body/spirit is vital to thriving.

#8 Be Visionary. Just like a little kid lying in the summer grass looking up to the sky imaging what could be, *Be Visionary* wants you to imagine your best life. With a bunch of tools to assist your visioning, including how to take your bad test results and make them work for you again, this chapter helps you create a new blueprint. If you've been feeling in a rut with your health, habits, and routine, *Be Visionary* gives you new lenses with which to see your world.

#9 Be Spontaneous. Being spontaneous can be streaking naked down the street or, as this chapter is about, the spontaneity that exists in each and every moment. You'll discover that getting the most from every moment is but a perception-shift away. We have to shed our preconceived ideas, our assumptions, about what will or won't happen, and allow the moment to unfold spontaneously.

#10 Be Limitless. Even if you diligently perfected the lessons in the previous nine chapters, if you leave your limitations in place, you'll only get so far. To shatter the barriers, *Be Limitless* has the tools you'll need to fully rejoice on another successful year. I want you to feel better than you may have ever imagined, so this chapter encourages you to go above and beyond, so that you can let go of the stress, and start to 'Be' you, uninhibited and super-charged, dynamic and free, moment after moment.

Chapter # 1 : Be Present

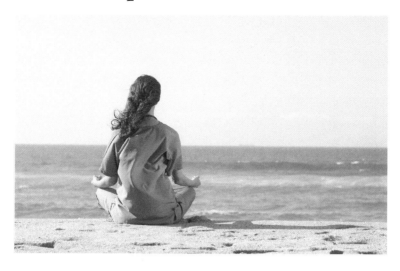

To mark the start of the darker half of the year, Celtic people celebrated the ancient festival of Samhain. A predecessor to 'Halloween', Samhain was believed to be a time to reevaluate, gather together and honor life and death. With celebrations to take stock of the past by listening to tales of the ancestors, honoring the present community, and to try to ensure the future safety of the departed, Samhain was believed to be a time when the veil between the worlds was lifted, allowing communication with the dead.

While we may not be conversing with the dead, the time has come to focus our energy on those parts of ourselves that have become lifeless, dull, uninspired, and exhausted. I see this regularly in my practice: legions of the walking wounded, shells of who people used to be, suffering the ills from the stress of the modern lifestyle. The perceived pressures have mounted higher and higher and eventually, our internal fire runs out of firewood and we become 'burnt out'.

Now is the time to reignite that fire, to unlearn those stressors, and set those old habits and stale thoughts afire. In their place, we will stoke the flames of desire and passion, cultivating a renewed zest for life.

The first step to this resurrection is the breath. In fact, this breath is the first and last step of life. Everything revolves around it. Your body needs it and

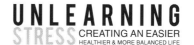

your spirit is elevated with it. Together, the back-and-forth of inhale and exhale kick-starts your transformation and is a constant barometer of your well-being.

This step is the most important part of your unlearning: your breath is more than you ever thought, or were taught, that it could be. Proper breathing is more than just a simple oxygen and carbon dioxide exchange. The breath is more than something you have to do to stay alive. Diaphragmatic breathing is something you must do in order to break the stress cycle and put your body in a position to truly thrive.

With one amazing breathe at a time, you can start to savor life. As you do this, your outlook will improve simply by the biochemical reaction deep breathing triggers. Deep breathing initiates a domino-like cascade of reactions throughout your entire body.

If you're thinking that I'm overstating the connection between breath and mind, try this: Imagine something that really scares you. Picture it in explicit and elaborate detail. If you're afraid of heights, mentally walk out onto the world's highest balcony.

> *"Breath is the bridge which connects life to consciousness,*
>
> *which unites your body to your thoughts."*
>
> *— Thich Nhat Hanh, Vietnamese monk, activist and writer*

Feel the wind racing past you, your knees becoming a little shaky, and then lean over a bit to see what the world looks like below. As you do, take in all that space between you and the cold, hard concrete below. Scary, huh?

Now, as you fixate on your fear, notice your posture. Your upper shoulders might have started to tense up and your body stiffen in preparation for (imaginary) battle. And your breathing? Probably pretty fast and shallow.

Now, banish those scary images from your mind and shift your focus onto something wonderful. Think of a place or activity that you love. Imagine the smells, the feelings on your skin, the people who are with you. As you begin

UNLEARNING STRESS CREATING AN EASIER HEALTHIER & MORE BALANCED LIFE

JAMES ROHR, L.Ac

to cherish this second scene, your breathing will also change. Again, notice your posture and your breathing and compare how different they are to the fear scenario.

How you are breathing tells you how you feel about your current environment and mindset. And by changing your breathing, you can change your experience of everything.

Breath is life and you are as good as the quality of your breath. Every major spiritual traditional incorporates some sort of breathing practice – meditation, chanting, and/or devotional singing- as one of the ways to become awake, aware, and fully conscious. "Throughout time the process of breathing was always considered inseparable from our health, consciousness, and spirit," notes Donna Farhi, yoga teacher, lecturer, and author of *The Breathing Book: Vitality and Good Health Through Essential Breath Work.*

While the breath can be a tool for incredible emotional and spiritual transformation, it starts with pressure changes in your lungs and the exchange of oxygen and carbon dioxide. To better understand this process, let's look at the anatomy. Below your ribcage is a dome-shaped muscle that extends from side to side called the thoracic diaphragm; above it reside your

Did You Know?

In Greek, psyche pneuma meant breath/soul/air/spirit. In Latin, anima spiritus, breath/soul, in Japanese, ki, air/spirit; and in Sanskrit, prana connoted a resonant life force that is at no time more apparent to us than when that force is extinguished at the moment of death. In Chinese the character for "breath" (hsi) is made up of three characters that mean of the conscious self or heart. The breath was seen as a force that ran through mind, body, and spirit like a river running through a dry valley giving sustenance to everything in its course.

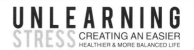

lungs and heart, and below which everything else can be found: the gall bladder, kidneys, liver, intestines, sex organs, and spleen. As the diaphragm moves up and down, the volume changes, and we experience breathing.

Although breathing is primarily governed by the diaphragm, other muscles are peripherally involved, including the intercostals muscles which move the ribs, as well as the scalenes, trapezius and pectoralis. If you've ever felt the weight of the world on your shoulders, these are some of the muscles we're talking about. If your shoulders are rounded forward, your head stuck forward like a turtle, and your chest feels tight, these are some of the muscles that shorten when struggling for breath. So, stop struggling with your breath and engage the diaphragm! With every deep, abdominal breath, the diaphragm comes in contact with several different organs. Energy is stimulated, the brain relaxes, and you feel better. But in case you're not sold, let's take a closer look:

FAST AND SHALLOW

aka stressed out, scared out your mind, breathing.

Instead of breathing primarily from your diaphragm, this kind of breathing involves a lot of the chest and accessory muscles, with very little movement of your abdomen. Your breathing here recruits the use of your scalenes and trapezius muscles. When your accessory muscles drive breathing, your breath automatically becomes much more rapid and shallow, which not only starts to limit the amount of oxygen being inhaled, but also cuts back on how much of the "waste product" – carbon dioxide – you're getting rid of when you exhale. Breathing like this for prolonged periods can also create or exacerbate neck tension. Chest-breathing quickly and shallowly tells your brain that your fight-or-flight flag is flying. This is your body saying it is feeling

Instead of your breath telling you how you feel about life, tell life how you feel about it by breathing it in to the fullest!

UNLEARNING STRESS CREATING AN EASIER HEALTHIER & MORE BALANCED LIFE

JAMES ROHR, L.Ac

threatened, which is not the message a happy, at-rest brain wants to hear.

SLOW AND DEEP

aka relaxing and lounging on a beach breathing

Great singers and babies have something important in common: they way they breathe. Singing well involves more than just innate talent; watch a great singer in action – their chest and abdomen seem to expand upward and outward, both front and back; babies, similarly breath in 3-D, as they inhale, their chubby little bellies rise and then collapse as they exhale. This type of breathing relies primarily on your diaphragm to inhale and exhale; as it contracts, the lower cavity pushes downward and because it is located next to your internal organs, this contracting/downward movement actually "massages" them.

Current research[1] shows that diaphragmatic breath training improves a number of functions: your lungs, immune system, the flow of lymph and blood, digestion, the onset and quality of sleep, reduces anxiety, blood pressure - and reduces pulmonary complications. Along with the kidneys, the liver, spleen and intestines are similarly squeezed and massaged, helping to purge stagnant energy and make room for the newly oxygenated blood to circulate more freely.

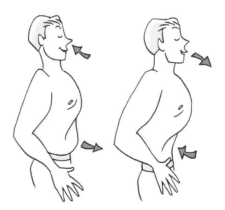

During the inhale, your heart maintains appropriate pressure in your chest by beating slightly faster; when you exhale, this same goal of

---

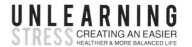

avoiding excessive pressure will actually cause your heart to beat slower, lowering your heart rate. Just by breathing out long and slow, you're having an immediate and positive impact on your heart rate and creating a more relaxed and healthy internal environment.[2] When your brain notes that you are breathing deeply, it interprets this to mean you are relaxed and at rest, so there must not be any imminent dangers – real or perceived – to worry about. When you breathe deeply, think of it as sending your brain happy news.

NOT BREATHING

Don't do this. Either you're in a dire situation, dead, almost dead, or super nervous/freaked out/scared out of your mind. In my years in clinic and lecturing about the breath and meditation, I've heard people over and over again say that they 'stop' breathing. They become aware during their breathing practice how often they hold their breath when they are stressed. Life is amazing, so let's savor it all with big, deep belly breaths.

> ## Quick Tip:
>
> *Inhale to a count of 4 seconds, hold it for 7 seconds, and exhale for 8 seconds. Give back a little more than you take in with every meditation breath.*

Not sure what kind of breathing you normally do? It's easy to tell the difference: if your chest moves up and down, then you're chest breathing; if your belly moves out and in then you are deep-belly breathing (like a balloon filling with air and then deflating).

Try this: place one hand on your stomach and the other on your chest. Now inhale. Did the hand on your abdomen move first? This is good sign. Even better if it moved out and in, rather than up and down. What about your top hand on your chest? Did it move at all? The less it moves the better, as it means you're breathing deeply and diaphragmatically.   Remember,

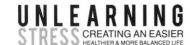

diaphragmatic breathing takes the load off those accessory upper-trapezius muscles where we all carry the weight of the world.

Every breath tells you how you are consciously/unconsciously feeling about the world. Every breath impacts your entire internal chemistry. Which way do you want to breathe? How do you want to live? Instead of your breath telling you how you feel about life, tell life how you feel about it by breathing it in to the fullest!

BE PRESENT

Try this:

In The Daily Relaxer: Relax Your Body, Calm Your Mind and Refresh Your Spirit,[3] authors Matthew McKay and Patrick Fanning note that "it only takes five or six deep breaths to begin reversing a tension spiral...As your diaphragm relaxes it sends an 'all's well' message to your brain, which becomes a signal for your whole body to release tension."

Deep Belly Breathing allows you to reduce the effects of stress in just a matter of a few breaths.

Close your eyes and inhale/exhale through your nose (if it's congested, then breathe however is comfortable)

Place one hand on your chest and the other on your stomach. Focus on keeping the chest hand still while your stomach moves slowly out and in, breathing into your back and outward with your abdomen.

As you exhale, purse your lips together as if you're about to blow out a candle, and try to make your exhale longer than your inhale. A Qi gong technique is to count to 4 as you inhale, then hold the breath for a count of 7, taking 8 to exhale. Each breath will probably last between 9 to 20 seconds; a fun goal is to see if you can slow it down to just 4-7 breaths/minute. Exaggerating the movement of your abdomen out and in and prolonging your exhale slows your heart rate, allows tension to escape your muscles and releases a lot more carbon dioxide.

When your cell or desk phone rings, don't answer it immediately. First take a moment to inhale, letting your abdomen expand. Exhale

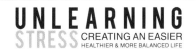

long and slow and then answer. Whenever you pour yourself – or buy - a fresh cup of coffee or tea, before that first sip, get in the habit of taking a deep breath. Use that breath as an opportunity to say a quick thanks; even if you're just expressing gratitude for the delicious drink in your hands. For extra credit, repeat before each sip. Deep Breath. Gratitude. Exhale. Sip. Enjoy. Repeat. And anytime you arrive at a parking space or even get into an elevator, take a deep breath first.

Set an hourly reminder on your cell to take a deep-breathing break.

READY FOR MORE? To really treat yourself to something sweet, try this mini breathing-getaway designed by Michelle Alva, a physical therapist, energy healer, and founder of *Nurturing Moves*[4]. When you have a minute to yourself, grab some pillows and lay down.

1. Lay on your back, the soles of your feet pressed together (your hips and thighs should flop open) or lay on your left side.

2. Place your pillows: Put one under your neck so that it stretches out and become parallel the surface you're laying on. If you're lying on your side, place another pillow between your legs so that your knees and ankles are parallel. Tuck yet another pillow under your right arm, allowing your shoulder, elbow and wrist to all become parallel.

3. Check your alignment: Your head, spine and pelvis should all be positioned neutrally. If need be, use more pillows until everything, your arms, your legs, every muscle, is ragdoll limp. "Positioning is very important to ensure maximum benefit and use of the right muscles to breathe," adds Michelle. "It is of utmost importance that we use the minimum amount of energy and optimal alignment of muscles during all exercises for our body to be able to prioritize healing."

4. Relax both your body and your mind, knowing that all this chillaxing is letting your breathing apparatus to function the way it was designed, which is returning the favor by helping you heal.

CUSTOMIZE: Learn from and revise your practice as you go along. Make some notes right after you do any breathing exercises. In your journal, take a minute or two to down how the practice was for you. Here are some questions to ask yourself to get your juices flowing:

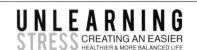

Did you remember to take deep breaths at the times you intended to? How did you feel afterwards?

Did you feel more relaxed or prepared to answer the phone, greet your family, respond to the email, etc.?

Have you experienced deeper breaths?

Are you noticing the tension in your abdomen releasing so that you can get even more expansion with each breath?

How many breaths are you averaging per minute? Try and slow it down without getting lightheaded.

ADD SOME SPICE

READ: *The Breathing Book: Vitality and Good Health Through Essential Breath Work* by Donna Farhi. Tips and techniques for unleashing the power of your most readily accessible resource.

LISTEN: *Breathing: The Master Key to Self-Healing* Audio CD by Andrew Weil, M.D. Eight exercises Weil uses in his own life and has also tested on hundreds of patients.

TRY: Rodney Yee's *Breathe: Relaxation and Breathing for Meditation (Audio).* Tips and tricks with spoken instruction and set to music.

EAT Lung-friendly foods include anti-inflammatory green tea, carrots for Vitamin A (great for fighting the toxins and pollution that like to live in the lungs), cold-water fish like salmon, mackerel, sardines and herring (Omega-3 fatty acids), Vitamin C (fruit, especially berries, and veggies like tomatoes)[5].

SMELL: Breathe in the deliciousness of life with some essential oils. I recommend the 6-oil sampler from Eden's Garden: Lavender (for calming) Eucalyptus (invigorating), Lemongrass (vitalizing and cleansing), Orange (uplifting), Peppermint (refreshing) and Tea Tree (purifying). And don't forget a diffuser!

BURN: Incense and fragrant herbs such as bundles of sage, cedar and sweet grass. Chinese medicine uses aromas to dissipate the fog of confusion and "heaviness" of the mind. By surrounding yourself with

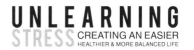

good smells, you're not just breathing more deeply, but you're using aromatherapy to help lift your mood and spirit.

Remember, you can't expect to feel vital and energized by shortchanging your body with shallow, rapid chest-breathing. One of the easiest most effective weapons at your disposal – whether you're a high-powered type with unlimited resources to spend on your health or on more of a budget – is learning to breathe, really breathe, and then start cultivating a regular deep-breathing practice. You may feel unusual or even uncomfortable at first, but give it time. In the beginning it may feel as though you can't get as deep breath as you can when you breathe with your chest, but it is just a matter of practice and allowing your abdominal muscles to relax that you will soon get a much deeper breath than was previously possible. Soon, you won't notice much chest involvement at all when you are doing this deep abdominal breathing. With a little more practice, you'll find this technique makes you feel relaxed, normal, and chill. Your discipline will pay off with more energy (more oxygen in the body), less neck and shoulder tension (you stop using them as the primary muscles for respiration), and ultimately more like a fully actualized version of you.

We can go days without food and water, yet only moments without air. Why not use some of those breaths as an opportunity to create movement in your abdomen, to release stagnant energy, and put the health odds in your favor. Deep breathing is cheap, portable, and readily available. All you have to do is remember to breathe this way until your body relearns relaxing breath and it becomes completely natural.

SUMMARY

Chapter 1: Be Present

- Deep Breathing is the cheapest, most accessible, and powerful tool for transforming your health and decreasing the stress response every moment.

- Stressed out breathing is shallow and vertical, with the neck and shoulders getting tight.

- To get the most relaxation and focus out of your breath make sure your abdomen expands on the inhale and contracts on the exhale

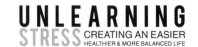

- For greater benefit during focused relaxation exercises, count to four on the inhale, hold it for five, and exhale for a count of six. Give back slightly more than you take in.

FOOD FOR THOUGHT FOR CHAPTER 1

What is your breathing saying about how you feel about life?

What are the times you find yourself holding your breath or doing shallow breathing? Do you notice a particular pattern among those times?

Why wouldn't you want to breathe in the most of this moment?

Can you pick something that you do often during the day and use that as a cue to do your deep breathing? What is it? Make a commitment to do it every day this week.

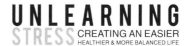

Chapter # 2 : Be Calm

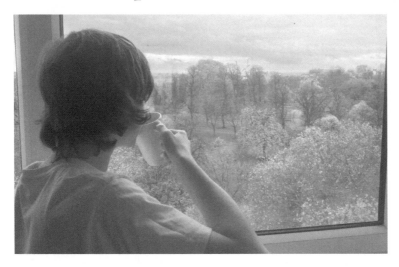

"In my hands, I hold a bowl of tea. Its green color is like a reflection of the nature surrounding us. I close my eyes and deep inside me, I see the green mountains and the clear spring water where it comes from. I am sitting by myself or with beloved ones, I am at peace and I feel that all this has become a part of me."

— Dr. Soshitsu Sen, Urasenke Grand Tea Master XV[6]

Since the year 727, when it was presented as a gift from the Chinese Tang court to Emperor Shomu, tea has been a part of Japanese culture. Although it was planted in the imperial garden in Kyoto around 794, it wasn't until 300 years later in 1191 when a Buddhist monk returned from China, planted tea seeds and wrote the book that influenced the development of the Japanese Tea Ceremony. Chanoyu , the Japanese Tea Ceremony ritual, has emerged as a moving meditation, combining art, spirituality, and community.

The setting of the tea ceremony is designed to help the participants retreat from the distractions of the regular world. "The intimate setting of the tea room, which is usually only large enough to accommodate four or five people, is modeled on a hermit's hut," explains the Metropolitan Museum of Art's Heilbrunn Timeline of Art History. "In this space, often surrounded by a garden, the participants temporarily withdraw from the mundane world."[7]

Every detail of the ceremony has been planned for and the aesthetic carefully chosen. From the ceramic tea bowls, the jars for water and vases for flowers, everything must lend itself to the full sensory enjoyment of the participants. The host is dutifully trained in everything from how to open the doors, how to walk, and of course, how to prepare the powdered green tea, matcha.

This elaborate choreography leads to an awakening of all the senses. When tea is served, the accompanying sound of the water, sight of the tea leaves, feel of the utensils, smell and taste of the tea bring your awareness into the present moment.[8] "What is learned in Chanoyu leads a person to the things in life that matter beyond the material things," notes Marjorie Yap, an accredited teacher from the Urasenke Chanoyu Institute in Kyoto, "and that is something that is enough for any lifetime."[9]

Cleansing of the senses to attain PURITY is one of the four main principles of the tea ceremony. The other three are: bringing oneself into HARMONY with others and nature, showing RESPECT, and cultivating TRANQUILITY.

Ritualizing the entire process of tea making and drinking has an amazing effect of quieting down our internal fight or flight system. If you're concerned about running for your life, your body won't be too concerned about enjoying the flavors of the tea you're trying to drink. There's no drive-thru tea ceremony! And during a regular day, do you know when you aren't going to be savoring all the subtle flavors of your food or drink? When you're stressed out, moving quickly, and scared out of your mind.

When you are in that fight or flight mode, a whole bunch of things are happening in the body to keep you upright and alive. As a trade-off, when this physiological system is active for a long time, it eventually doesn't offer a whole lot when it comes to enjoying the finer things in life.

In our not-so-distant past, we survived by foraging for food, hunting, and probably the most important skill of all: the ability to avoid getting killed.

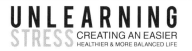

How? By being able to respond quickly or haul ass to safety at a moment's notice. Should a bear or other predator suddenly materialize, our internal resources were mobilized by two teensy walnut-shaped glands situated just above the kidneys. The adrenals secrete messenger molecules, called hormones, including cortisol and epinephrine, aka adrenaline, to travel through the bloodstream and tell other body parts what to do.

Being awash in adrenaline facilitates a number of escape-the-threat defenses: it dilates your eyes (the better to see everything), makes blood more available for ass-hauling by speeding up the heart rate and sending the blood pressure into orbit. In combination, all these reactions combine to help you answer the following at lightening, hopefully life-saving speed:

Should I try and flee or stay and fight for my life?

The flight-or-fight response is, obviously, an extreme response to a clear and present danger; its "command center" is the sympathetic nervous system (SNS). Since SNS is devoted to saving your life, when activated, it automatically becomes top priority and temporarily overrides every other function. However, once the threat has passed, your SNS need no longer remain on high alert, so the DEFCON signals can chill out.

Once the SNS is "off", its counterpart, the parasympathetic nervous system (PNS) can then turn back "on" and return things to normal (or what used to be normal before Westerners became stressed out all the time that they have forgotten what relaxed feels like). The PNS calms your fast-beating heart, slows down your breathing and facilitates proper digestion and elimination.

"So what," we hear you thinking. "The adrenaline rush and SNS is automatic and natural. Why would it be harmful?"

I'm so glad you asked.

> *Can't keep SNS and PNS straight?*
>
> *Think of the first S as Scared, or S.O.S distress calls*
>
> *P in PNS as Peaceful and Playful.*

UNLEARNING STRESS CREATING AN EASIER HEALTHIER & MORE BALANCED LIFE

JAMES ROHR, L.Ac

What started off as a life-saving first alert system in response to obvious threats to life and limb – bears, lions and the like – has not evolved in tandem with our environment. The threats under which our SNS developed were real, but extremely short-lived. Either the bear got you or your number wasn't quite up and you made it to safety. The SNS was adapted to this short burst of outdoor activity. However, as we came indoors, the threats changed. We now have imaginary bears and lions and tigers constantly piling into our thoughts, emails, and text messages 24/7. So our short term distress system is no longer short; it is never allowed to scale back.

Our nervous system stays on high alert as it tries to protect us from impending doom. When this system does damage, it does so because it is going on for far too long. The good news is we can change it, if we stop seeing ourselves as constantly in danger. Because if we always feel threatened, the SNS activity will continue for years and years without end until one day, your entire body breaks down.

Most people are not actually in life threatening situations anymore. So what are people spending so much of the time feeling the need to protect? There is something we have that is very fragile and is on guard like a jealous lover: our egos. This ego, this thing that feels the need to be special, differentiated, loved, and adored, is keeping us on high alert. And it is completely unnecessary.

Part of this process of healing and transforming, of shifting out of a perceived life and death situation, involves being able to see beyond the lenses of our ego. Let's take a look at some of the common, though often unspoken, threats to the ego that can activate the SNS…:

> …being embarrassed or humiliated in front of your peers.
>
> …not getting that promotion.
>
> …being perceived as not good enough or a total failure.
>
> …having unrealistic expectations of yourself,
>
> …scrambling to meet a tough deadline.
>
> …having a To Do list that never ends.
>
> …getting stuck in traffic.
>
> …problems with money and finances.

 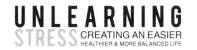

…arguing with your partner.

…getting laid off or fired.

In addition to these ego-related bogeymen, we often self-sabotage with food, grabbing junk instead of nourishment, and either not exercising enough or being an exercise addict. These dubious choices have dubious consequences such as:

…blood sugar crashes and surges

…eating foods you're intolerant or allergic to.

…exercising to the point of over-training.

…having intestinal issues,

…internal inflammation.

> *The threats that cause most of the damage are NOT actually life threatening anymore.*

Now a little stress response isn't a bad thing per se – it's designed to be higher first thing in the morning to motivate you to wake up and get going, and then taper off so that at bedtime, you're sleepy. However, when this natural rhythm is disrupted and cortisol not only stays elevated, but there's more of it, it may:

…raise your blood sugar, making you hungry and crave sugar.

…make your gut leaky.

…reduce your ability to burn body fat.

…weaken your immune system

…unbalance your hormone levels,

…make your moody, anxious and even depressed.

…contribute to heart disease.

The problem with keeping your SNS "on" all the time is that when it's operational, PNS must be off; and vice versa; they cannot both be fully active in the same organ at the same time. If your chronic state of stress keeps your SNS permanently "on", guess what isn't getting its chance to repair and relax you back to vibrant health? Exactly. Your PNS.

UNLEARNING
STRESS CREATING AN EASIER
HEALTHIER & MORE BALANCED LIFE

If you had carpal tunnel pain from typing, you'd need to change something or your hands may not be able to heal. Similarly, if you react to your job, or life, with heart palpitations, unless you change how you perceive the stress it will continue to compromise your heart. Just because you can't put a Band-Aid on the injury or see the damage being done does not mean everything is okay. If you're feeling unhealthy and threatened, the time for change is now.

Constant stimulation of the SNS contributes to the creation and development of illness. The physiological changes occurring on a cellular level are not sustainable. The body is never given any downtime and allowed to heal, so damaged cells continue to replicate unchecked, inflammation grows, and hormones are unbalanced. Without intervention, this illness will continually be created and worsened as the body becomes more and more unable to regulate itself.

Even threats that are perceived or imaginary are acted upon the same by your body.

This may look like an S.O.S. in the form of "chronic illness," be it fatigue, difficulties falling and/or staying asleep, constant headaches, digestive distress, or extreme moodiness.

Not all illness is a result of an overactive SNS, but in terms of quality of life and our activities of daily living, an overactive SNS is usually culprit #1. Even Chinese medicine, thousands of years ago, has noted that stress is a cause of disease. What I have found in my study and practice of this medicine is that what Chinese medicine says is enough stress to cause disease is what the average Westerner considers normal day-to-day operations. So when a Westerner says they're stressed out, the threat is off-the-charts dangerous.

Remember: even threats that are perceived or imaginary are acted upon the same by your body. In fact, the threat from a predator is probably less damaging because it's limited to a short burst of time; a deadline, however, is a threat that is sustained for days, weeks or months. Outrun or outsmart the predator and the threat of death recedes, allowing your body to recover. On the other hand, your SNS will continue to remain active as long as the deadline looms until you feel totally frazzled and fried. Adrenaline is pumped thru the body and PNS is never allowed to re-stock the shelves of our relaxing and healing chemicals.

And while you can't control your pupils dilating or your heart contracting more rapidly, the switch which turns these processes on is within your control. You have the power to slow down or stop a cascade. If you've been practicing Chapter #1, Be Present, you've already started to bring balance to your body because prolonged exhalation stimulates the Vagus nerve, activating the PNS. The key is to make stress management something you assign a high priority to and, like bathing and brushing your teeth, something you just do every day.

How?

Although some "stress" is good, helping to keep you stimulated, engaged and active, your body does need sufficient PNS activity to recover at the cellular level. If you want to feel your most vibrant and healthy, then know that this recovery is mandatory. There are a number of different options which are worth checking out until you discover one you really love and can stick with for the long run.

DEFUSE THE WORRY BOMB

If you have kept your SNS running in constant overdrive to the point where it's an automatic habit, learning to "cope" with stress - be it rest, medication, exercise, denial, talk therapy, or even substance abuse – is like a Band-Aid covering a wound: temporary. Temporary help is better than no help, but let's go another step further.

Why just cope when you can defuse the loaded situation altogether?

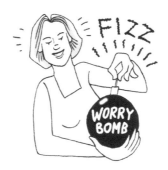

UNDERSTAND SNS'S POINT OF VIEW

Most likely, whatever is stressing you out is not a physical threat to your survival. How many truly life-threatening situations have you been in recently? Getting stuck in traffic, missing a phone call, or even missing a deadline, rarely results in an actual loss of life. But, responding to any of these so called threats by being stressed out activates that life-threatening response. The farmer having a hard time because of drought and lack of crops experiences the same stress in response in the body as the suburban housewife who is mortified about what "people might think". Because it can't tell the difference between the "real" threat and the one that is perceived, the SNS will activate in either situation. *The key thing to understand about the SNS is that it does not discriminate between threats.*

CHANGE YOUR PERCEPTION

Once you understand that stress results in the same response, it becomes obvious that you have a few choices. One might be able to change jobs or make lifestyle tweaks; on a deeper level, it might be time to change how you perceive a "threat" so that you're not forcing your body to constantly mobilize the fight-or-flight defense system. Some of the way you perceive threats isn't actually your fault! Rather, it's cultural programming: "We experience stress because of the meaning we assign to certain events or situations," says Chris Kresser, an acupuncturist and radio host. "For example, being stuck in traffic can be a "disaster" or it could be an opportunity for contemplation and solitude."[10] Deadlines only matter if you care about meeting them.

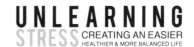

TAILOR YOUR RESPONSE

Once you start to distinguish between types of threats, you'll want to work on unlearning the responses which add to your stress levels. You will begin to embrace reactions that bring you back in line with health. Change your mind and change how your body responds. Just think: that very same stressor that yesterday made you want to throttle someone may suddenly lose its power. Instead of being sucked into a wormhole of rage and frustration, you may find that you can simply shrug your shoulders and mentally move on. Start examining your expectations from certain situations, yourself, and your lifestyle. If you find old habits hard to kill, don't be discouraged; your thoughts that are causing so much damage can be changed, one moment at a time.

Think of certain situations that get you fired up. Write down how you responded and then **write down how you would ideally respond.** As you continue thru these chapters, return to this list to remind you where you need to be extra vigilant in your life and to give you an image of your ideal attitude.

The mind, and our automatic responses, behaves just like a puppy that needs training. Without clear boundaries, the puppy, and mind, will tend to pee and poop everywhere. By being vigilant observers of ourselves, and applying consistent direction and boundaries, we re-train our responses. And then you

About Worrying

So much of what triggers our worry is stuff that happened before or stuff that is happening outside of your control. Worry is using your imagination to create what you don't want. Rather than dwell with the worry, use your imagination towards what you do want. Spend your worry time towards visualizing what you do want instead of what you don't want. Why drown in the past or an imagined, horrible future when the present moment is unfolding so peacefully right now?

start to realize that you do have the ability to control the things your mind tends to dwell on. This is when your mind will stop "pooping" in the living room and understand how you want to behave.

MAKE LITTLE CHANGES

In dangerous situations, your SNS response is invaluable, so the goal is not to disable it completely. Rather, focus on disrupting thinking that sees stress and pressure around every corner, despite the fact there isn't any impending threat to your physical survival. For maximum health and a sustainable transformation, the goal is to balance time spent in SNS with PNS.

What little changes can you make to spend more in the PNS (hint: the chapters in this book!)? Write them down in your journal. I suggest starting with making a commitment to do the deep breathing exercises throughout the day.

WORRY YOUR WAY TO HAPPY

Caution: this next step is the worrying equivalent of locking yourself in a closet with a carton of cigarettes. This approach can have some heavy consequences, and puts the body in a bit of frenzy with the goal of overloading and 'short circuiting' the worrying hotline.

For this step, I suggest to get your worry on for 5 full minutes, especially everything you normally worry about and stress over throughout the day. Set your timer for 5 minutes and then worry, worry and worry some more. Allow yourself to get worked up, overwrought, anxious and full-on stressed. Relish this time to worry. Go ahead, marinate in it! Give yourself full permission to get your worrywart on.

When the timer goes off, you're done. Absolutely no more worrying allowed for the rest of the day. During the rest of the day, anytime you notice you're over-reaching or worrying, make a quick note to yourself in your gadget or notebook about whatever triggered your worry or what you're obsessing over. Once you've written it down, do your best to forget about it until tomorrow's worry session, when you should feel free to refer liberally to your notes. Tip: Don't cut your sanctioned-worry time short; be sure to take full advantage of your five-minute worry fest because when the timer goes off, you're no longer allowed to worry until the next day. The key is using the full five minutes of worry time; this oversaturation helps to really drive the point home that worrying and overreacting is harmful.

The purpose of this awareness is to give your mind a place to feel free to react/over-react. Then, by clearly establishing some boundaries, you realize that no one has power over your emotional state but you. Saying "s/he made me feel _____" is inaccurate. The reality is you chose to feel how you felt based on a certain stimulus. Or, perhaps more accurately, you chose to dwell on certain thoughts or feelings long past the initial stimulus happened. The initial thoughts are based on incredibly rapid firing of neurons, but how you respond to that firing is something you can control. If you believe you can't control it, then you never will. You will continue to be at the mercy of how the environment and the people around you treat you. That isn't a very empowered place to be. Don't be fooled by the myth that stress and worry will help you succeed. It won't. Overreacting, and needless worry, leads to fatigue, lack of clarity and bad decisions; it actually disrupts success. In other words, continuing to worry and stress is both a waste of your time and your health.

ADD SOME SPICE

READ: *Why Zebras Don't Get Ulcers* by Robert Sapolsky

LISTEN: BREATHING: *The Master Key to Self-Healing* Audio CD by Andrew Weil, M.D. Eight exercises Weil uses in his own life and has also tested on hundreds of patients.

DO: Deepak Chopra's system, *Wild Divine*, is a great tool for biofeedback. With relaxation techniques, biofeedback adventures, and meditations, this computer based system makes this training fun

FEEDBACK: Other biofeedback machines can also be very helpful to help retrain your physiologic response. HeartMath is an incredible company that is doing a lot of research into how better to understand our biorhythms and gain control of our reactions. Their product, *emWave2*, is a great at-home device that gives you real-time feedback on your internal heart rhythms so you can experiment to see which techniques, thoughts, breathing exercises, etc. help you quiet yourself down the most quickly. With digital displays on your computer, this device helps to externalize your inner reactions.

GET: Acupuncture. This 3,000+ year old system is amazing at activating the PNS and decreasing the SNS response. Whether you need to completely reboot your energy or just give your nervous system a mini-vacation, it's incredible how even one 45 minute acupuncture session can have long term benefits on your body and mind's ability to overcome stress. Check out *www.nccaom.org* to find a licensed acupuncturist in your area.

Instead of allowing yourself to feel frustrated – at a situation, at your body, at your symptoms –realize that feeling frustrated blocks the flow of your energy. When you can take a deep breath, get some perspective, and allow the PNS to help you get grounded, amazing things can start happening. You find that you are not at the mercy of everything around you anymore. This means that then you are better able to dictate how you are going feel, or react to your feelings. Some physical symptoms may remain or may need further intervention, but choosing not to be at the mercy of everything around you (your diagnosis, family, job, etc.) is true empowerment, and freedom from the enslavement of stress and your SNS spiral.

SUMMARY

Chapter 2: Be Calm

- There are two major nervous systems in the body: 'the 'oh shit, fight or flight system' and the 'ah, nice, resting and relaxing system.'

- The majority of healing occurs when the body is in the resting and relaxing system

- Where the fight or flight system used to be active for only brief periods of time, we are now seeing this system being activated almost all the time. This is leading to exhaustion, burnout, anxiety, panic attacks, and more.

- In order to spend more time in the relaxing mode, we have to defuse our internal fears triggered by the should, would, could, past, or future focus.

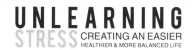

FOOD FOR THOUGHT FOR CHAPTER 2

When do you feel threatened? Make a list of the triggers for your fight or flight reactions. Throughout the day, notice and write down the triggers. Is it work? Being late? Not being good enough? Was your life actually in immediate danger?

Write down where and when you get triggered. This is the process of discovering yourself so you can make conscious change. How did you respond when you felt threatened? Was this response how you would want to respond all the time? Or is there another way you want to respond?

What are three small changes you can make to decrease these triggers?

Which triggers can you eliminate?

How else can you make changes to strengthen your resolve?

UNLEARNING STRESS CREATING AN EASIER HEALTHIER & MORE BALANCED LIFE

JAMES ROHR, L.Ac

Chapter #3 : Be Seated

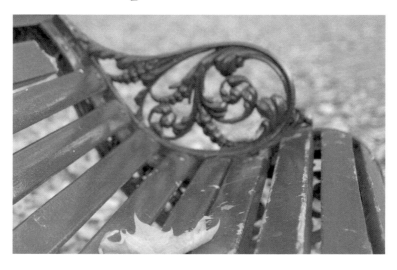

"Ten thousand flowers in spring the moon in autumn, a cool breeze in summer, snow in winter. If your mind isn't clouded by unnecessary things, this is the best season of your life."

— Wu-men Hui-k'ai, 13th century[11]

Let your mind meander back to a day you really enjoyed.

Immerse yourself in the scene, feeling the air on your skin, taking note of the weather, whoever is with you, and whatever you're doing that is so much fun. Now, imagine you get an urgent text. It's your accountant (*sigh*). Bad news: 30% of the value of your retirement savings is gone. How do you respond?

In an ideal world:

> "I've been having such a great day. I notice I responded with thoughts of being afraid and anxious, and angry of course, but my immediate survival isn't in jeopardy. I know there's a solution, an answer. And right now, what would make me feel best is to continue enjoying my day."

Okay, now let's get real:

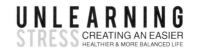

"Oh my god, my money is gone! What do I do? Who's to blame for this?!"

The default go-to position for most of us is automatically fear, which is why the first response sounds ridiculous, the second believable. Every time you receive news, or perceive a situation, that means you will lose, the mechanical, or unconscious, way to respond is the way you always have a gazillion times before: panic, dread, anger, fear. Regardless of what you struggle with, from finances to friendship to the family, when we find ourselves in situations we don't like or receive news we consider bad, we react. The same way. Every time. Just like with mechanical robots: push this button=expected thing happens; push this emotional button = the same emotional outcome.

Rather than experiencing the moment, we zoom ahead to the future ("oh now, my savings are gone – what will become of me?") or run for the safety-blanket of the past ("this always happens to me, I'm such a loser!"). What we rarely do: simply be, without judging the inputs. The problem with living in the future or the past is that it alienates us from our lives as they happen.

Can we break our damaging habits of mechanical behavior and over-reactions?

Actually, yes.

Here's how:

For the next 30 seconds, close your eyes and focus on your breath going in and out of your nose. Make a note of how the air feels on your skin (is it hot? freezing?), any sounds you hear, what you smell and the taste in your mouth. Just experience them. If you start making judgments about any of this ("oh wow, listen to that siren, there must be an accident" or "I'm cold, I should probably put a sweater on") simply make a note about what these thoughts are and then let them be.

> *The problem with living in the future or the past is that it alienates us from our lives as they happen.*

Then open your eyes. Congratulations, you just employed a simple but amazingly effective weapon in your health arsenal: you meditated.

By focusing on your senses, did you notice any thoughts that meandered away from the present moment? By *noticing*, and not fixating, on those thoughts, you did something really important during your mini meditation session: you put yourself in the now. And now is where life's magic is happening. "We only have moments in which to live," notes author and meditation expert Jon Kabat-Zinn. "The future is a concept; the past, memory, is a concept; but the only time in which our lives are unfolding is now."[12] Living in the present means treating every moment with equal regard and experiencing all of them fully.

Over time, as you practice, you will be able to stave off such melodrama by sitting quietly and attending to the present moment. You can allow yourself to fully experience your feelings, taking notice of whatever you think, but without having to judge your thoughts or be owned by them. The key is to observe yourself and notice where your mind may wander, but to no longer be ruled by your thoughts. With mindfulness, you can become less of a dandelion in the wind and more like a windmill, harnessing the power of your mind to help you feel your best.

So, what are you paying attention to in this mindfulness practice? Discover your conditioning, the stuff you like and don't like, your judgments and burdens, the stuff you feel you should/shouldn't/would/could/have to do or have done. Eventually, you can delete those thought files that are inconsistent with the life you want to be living. You will arrive at a more authentic, spontaneous, and compassionate way of being. This awareness limits the amount of time SNS is in control, giving PNS the chance to cultivate an internal environment that promotes healing. The keys are practice and diligence.

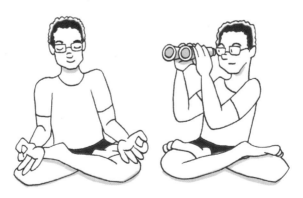

UNLEARNING STRESS CREATING AN EASIER HEALTHIER & MORE BALANCED LIFE

Use this meditation time to begin to see you, to watch yourself through different lenses. Offer some of the parts of yourself you don't like some metaphorical wine and cheese. Invite those less likeable parts of yourself to come and feast with you so you can get to know all of you. From this awareness, you begin to come from an empowered place. You've gathered all the information about various stimuli. You see what has motivated you and what works or doesn't work well. All of this can come from being seated and watching without judgment.

You may see that part of yourself driven to climb the corporate ladder, diligently powering through your never-ending To Do list, complete all the various tasks you've set yourself because that's what you think you need to do. You may see yourself reacting to all those ego involved thoughts from the Chapter 2. You may even watch yourself trying to meditate correctly, to do it the 'right' way. But all this doing-doing-doing comes at a cost. We continually operate at less than our potential.

Cultivating mindful awareness is the way to gain control of what you think and how you react. Think this is impossible? In the military, soldiers are trained in mindful awareness. They reprogram their physiological responses to dire situations in order not to be at the mercy of their instincts; instincts which may be shouting at them to run from danger. Instead of their instincts making decisions for them, the soldiers consciously decide. And in that process of conscious decision making, they train their body to behave how they need it to in times of crisis.

> *Often times it is not the actual symptoms that squeeze the joy out of life; rather, it is our reaction to the symptoms.*

When we are sick, we may have to re-train our reactions to this crisis. I have seen that many of the reactions that impede our quality of life are directly related to our specific illnesses and imbalances. It is bad enough to have back pain, but to be angry at yourself because you can no longer over-extend yourself to be super-parent makes it even worse. The same is true for women who are infertile and think they 'should' be pregnant or that they are failing their partners by not being able to get pregnant. It can be hard enough to conceive, and adding the stress of the extra story doesn't help. Often times, it is not the actual symptoms that squeeze the joy out of life, rather, it is our reaction to them. Combining the breath with clarity of awareness regarding what is a threat and what isn't, puts you back on the throne overseeing the kingdom that is your life.

Once you have your breathing practice underway (Chapter #1) and have started to reframe how you react to various situations (Chapter #2), you can then nudge your overall health even further in the right direction just by starting to pay attention to what's going through your head. Not only will you be able to better control reactions that automatically trigger your SNS, but you'll be helping give the PNS its fair time in the ring, which will allow it to restore and optimize your health, including your immunity. Your immune system is heavily influenced by the ever-changing mosaic in your mind and study after study has shown that under stress, the body's immunity is weakened, including "natural killer cell activity" which is thought to "play an important role in the body's defense mechanisms against cancer and viral infections," adds Kabat-Zinn in his wonderful book *Full-Catastrophe Living*.[13]

If we do no additional harm and get out of the way, the body is generally the best doctor there is. Interestingly, all this sitting around and "being" can actually profoundly improve the health of your brain. Researchers at UCLA discovered that the longer someone had meditated, the more "folding" (gyrification) there was in the cortex area that may allow for faster processing of information and better ability to form memories, maintain attention and consciousness and adapt to change (neuroplasticity). "Meditators are known to be masters in introspection and awareness as well as emotional control and self-regulation," noted one of the researchers, "so the findings make sense that the longer someone has meditated, the higher the degree of folding in the insula [a hub for thought, consciousness, processing info and making decisions]."[14]

Meditation has also been shown to increase out-of-the-box creative thinking,[15] make it easier to concentrate[16] for longer periods of time in a more discerning fashion,[17] help with insomnia and sleep issues,[18] lower blood pressure[19] and the risk of heart disease,[20] and reduce the emotional impact of chronic pain[21] which is often accompanied by depression.

And you won't even have to wait years to experience many of these benefits. Try weeks, even as few as five – with as little as two 30-minute sessions a week - as one study at the University of Wisconsin discovered. "If someone is thinking about trying meditation and they were thinking, 'It's too big of a commitment, it's going to take too much rigorous training before it has an effect on my mind,' this research suggests that's not the case," notes one of the researchers, adding that for those people, meditation might be worth a try. "It can't hurt and it might do you a lot of good."[22]

BE SEATED

Left to please itself, your mind will react to situations in ways that will lead to robotic behavior. The most effective way to combat this conditioning is with some discipline. How? Just like training your body when working out you can train your mind by sitting. So why do I call it sitting instead of meditation? Mostly because meditation is a loaded term that brings up all sorts of preconceived ideas and fear from the over-committed, busy American. But whether you call it meditating or the more ordinary, sitting, they are merely different terms for the same activity: paying attention.

There are so many ways to meditate and practice mindfulness, some of which go beyond sitting to include movement based exercise, like yoga, tai chi, or qi gong. Below are a few suggestions for more seated practices that can hopefully carry over into your day to day. For practice you'll need somewhere to sit quietly and make some time for yourself. Some of these suggested practices can be used by themselves or combined with other ones. There is no right or wrong here. The point is to discover yourself so you can feel healthier, more alive, and free. But remember, this is just practice. The goal is to make your life your meditation, so one day you can be as mindfully aware while stuck in traffic as you are in your meditation parlor.

TAKE A LOOK AROUND

Don't worry about pretzeling up into the lotus position or lounging on special floor-cushions. In fact, don't "do" anything other than look around and listen actively. You needn't worry about "clearing" your mind; rather, observe and listen. As you hear sounds, when you start guessing and jumping to conclusions about what's causing them, stop yourself. For example, if you

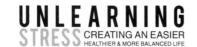

hear a siren, don't assume it's from an ambulance possibly coming from the scene of an accident and zooming to a hospital; instead, just notice how the siren sounds and any changes in loudness as it comes nearer and then moves away.

WHY: This practice is designed to make you accustomed to using your senses to shut down the filters you've made, your assumptions and preferences, and allow yourself to experience the present moment in full.

FOCUS ON YOUR NOSE, SEE WHAT'S ON YOUR MIND

Spend some time in a seated practice with your entire awareness on the tip of your nose. You don't have to close your eyes, but it can help to focus the mind. Let other sensations fade away and focus on your breathing. Follow your breathing in and out. At some point, your mind will probably wander, and when it does, make a brief observation of where it goes.

WHY? Every time you think about stuff other than the tip of your nose and your breathing, that's okay – it's a good way to really understand not only what's on your mind, but just how hyperactive you mind it. Where does your mind go? Does it go to the same place/person/thing over and over and over again? Often times making lasting change isn't the hard part, it is the recognizing that a change needs to be made in the first place. Observe the places or people your mind travels to without judgment. When your meditation practice time is over, you'll have plenty of time to process your thoughts and strategize how to create more freedom in your mind and heart.

> *Often times making lasting change isn't the hard part, it is the recognizing that a change needs to be made in the first place. Observe the places or people your mind travels to without judgment.*

NO 'DOING' ALLOWED

Just be yourself. You are a unique combination of energy that at its core is like an internal fire. Rediscover your passion for life and quite possibly enjoy yourself without needing any extra stimulation or action plans to accomplish created goals or accomplishments. Just be. Can you imagine a world where this is your only responsibility? I hope so because this is your greatest responsibility in the world: be yourself.

WHY: Having a To Do list of stuff you want to accomplish from meditating – from getting better/faster/stronger to unraveling a Gordian knot of problems – defeats the very purpose. No one is grading you on your performance and you can't 'beat' or 'win' the meditation game.

TUNE IN

Plan to sit quietly for at least 5 minutes. Check in with yourself to see how you are feeling, what you're thinking, do you like what you're thinking, and are you living the life you want to be living? If having meaningful relationships is important to you, how can you offer anything meaningful if you don't know what you mean? Use this mindfulness to check-in and recalibrate to your highest levels of being.

WHY? A formal meditation practice, even if it's just for 30 seconds, will help you to start to tune you into the bigger symphony that's playing your life's song. You can think of sitting as similar to what the members of a symphony orchestra do before they play – they make sure their instruments are in tune and attuned to each other. Otherwise, the resulting performance suffers. "It would be like a great symphony orchestra playing Beethoven without tuning first," says Kabat-Zinn. "No matter if they have the greatest musicians or greatest instruments in the world, you still tune first – to themselves and to each other. In some sense, you could say meditation is like tuning your instrument before you take it out on the road. And tuning it in the morning can make a big difference with how the whole day goes."

GET COMFY WITH BEING UNCOMFY

However you choose to do your attention paying, be it cross-legged and enveloped in incense and Sanskrit, on an elaborate vision quest, in a sweat

UNLEARNING STRESS CREATING AN EASIER HEALTHIER & MORE BALANCED LIFE

lodge, or simply sitting quietly, an important skill to develop is your ability to sit for long stretches, especially if it's a bit uncomfortable.

WHY: Being able to sit for a spell while uncomfortable teaches your mind time to get used to processing unpleasant experiences without "running away". Ditto sitting with chronic pain as sometimes your body just needs to experience pain. Learning to sit, regardless of how boring it may feel, you start to become aware of how much of your life is devoted to chasing something as illusory as 'comfort'. We try to create a life without too many variables so we are as non-disturbed as possible. If we learn to embrace disturbances, we open ourselves up to enjoying a lot more of what life has to offer.

BORE YOURSELF SILLY

Five minutes of sitting is good, but 30 is even better – especially if you start to get antsy and really bored.

WHY? From the Chinese medicine world, we need to cultivate more yin, the quiet, calming, soothing, grounded energy to help offset the extroverted, energizing, erratic, chaotic yang energy. Our western culture cherishes this preponderance of yang while trying to ignore the importance of the yin practice. Take your time, try to enjoy the stillness while your body absorbs and creates this yin energy. Think of yang as the fire and the yin as the firewood. Quiet, slow, calming practices help to replenish the yin. Without it, eventually the fire starts to go out.

When you get 'bored', you begin to see how much yang energy you use all day. You see how you crave that energy. Just think how much yin energy you need to counteract all that yang you put into your life to keep from feeling bored.

THOUGHTS=LESSONS

This is soooooooo boring. I hate this meditation stuff…what nonsense. My butt hurts. I'm thirsty. I wonder how long I've been meditating? It probably won't take too long before this simple assignment of watching your breath proves way easier said than done. Thoughts creep in. Don't fight them or berate yourself for being a crappy meditator. Instead, welcome them when they appear.

WHY? People expect meditation to be calming and easy, but often times in the beginning it is like shaking a snow globe. You sit and the mind is shaken and thoughts start swirling everywhere; thoughts you may not have even been aware of because they had 'settled' into the ground. Now that you're sitting, everything is getting shaken up.

One of the biggest misconceptions about meditating is believing that it's about making your mind blank and shutting off your thinking. However, thoughts are actually part of the curriculum. They teach us where we are distracted in our lives. The invasive thoughts show us where we may be leaking emotional and physical energy. From this awareness, after our meditation practice, we will be able to focus on remedies and solutions for these distractions. The result is a cleaner, simpler life with fewer bottomless pits of anxiety trying to pull us in.

We are in the habit of distracting ourselves: I wonder if I have any new email since the last time I checked (30 seconds ago)? What's happening on Facebook? What is on television? We've become masters of deceiving ourselves, telling ourselves that something "important" might be at stake. We're trying to distract ourselves out of having to experience the current moment exactly the way it is. Because we may realize that the now isn't as good as we had hoped. When you sit, you start to deal with the suggestions and lies you tell yourself. Taking the risk to be present, you will become less afraid. And a person unafraid of themselves is a person unafraid to experience spontaneous love.

STAY AWAKE

One of the "occupational hazards" of meditating is falling asleep on the job. If you're chronically sleep-deprived, do more sleeping and less meditating until you start to get caught up. However, once you're more rested, if you still find yourself dozing off, ask yourself: how motivated am I to stay awake while meditating?

WHY: If you've ever driven at night and dozed off at the wheel, you probably rolled down the windows, blasted the radio, and maybe even smacked yourself – whatever it took. The consequences of not being awake were dire enough that you were highly motivated to stay awake. Similarly, with meditation, are you willing to think creatively, possibly sitting uncomfortably, changing the time you meditate, and maybe even taking a cold shower first? Ultimately, this practice is a metaphor for your life. Do you want to sleep thru your life or are you willing to stay awake, stay alert, and pay attention?

EXTEND YOUR MINDFULNESS INTO YOUR DAY

Conclude your formal meditation by setting an intention for yourself, maybe something as simple as being nice to someone or taking more deep breaths throughout the day. When you're walking the dog, simply experience the moment: watch the dog enjoying itself, feel the air on your skin, the sounds around you. Even if you're just sweeping the floor, look at the handle of the broom. Is it plastic or made from wood? New or worn? Rough or smooth? When you hold it, how does it feel in your hands? How about your shoulders – how do they feel as you move back and forth?

WHY: Being present and accounted for in your life means cutting back on zone-out time as much as possible and being here now. If you find your day is filled with situation after situation where you'd rather not be present, perhaps it's time to ask yourself if this is the life you want to be living. If not, then what do you want? Start to become an active partner in the dance that is your life.

Instead of being lost in thought, be present in your life. Tell your mind and body to "stay put" so you can be present with your kids or partner instead of answering the phone or checking email. Your goal is to eventually be present more often than not, making your day one long, blissful meditation.

ADD SOME SPICE

WATCH: *Mindfulness with Jon Kabat-Zinn* (YouTube video). Kabat-Zinn specializes in helping people cope with stress, anxiety, pain and illness. A molecular biologist with a Ph.D. from Massachusetts Institute of Technology (MIT), he is the author of myriad books on the topic, including *Wherever You Go, There You Are* and founder of the Stress Reduction Clinic and Center for Mindfulness in Medicine, Health Care and Society at the University of Massachusetts Medical School.

BUY: Noise-canceling headphones. If quieting your mind is proving really challenging, try blocking out ambient noise, additional sounds and feedback around you with noise-canceling headphones. The Bose ones rock, but any high-quality ones will help give you a high(er) quality sitting session. Just think of it as better meditation through technology. Especially when you combine with the next suggestion.

TRY: Getting your sonic experience on. Your moods are correlated with four main categories of brainwaves. When you're chillaxing or awake but relaxing with your eyes closed, your Alpha brainwaves dominate. Being focused, energized and busy relies on Beta brainwaves while being creative or going into a deep meditative state relies on Theta waves. And sleep is most often associated with Delta waves. To consciously switch between states, try a brainwave-activating CD or DVD which switches inputs between the left and right hemispheres, influencing the brainwaves. They are most effective when used with headphones.

The Brainwave Symphony by Jeffrey Thompson, a pioneer in the field, is particularly excellent. "A good part of the stress we all experience… is due to the advancements of our own technology," notes Thompson. "This same technology, combined with our traditional techniques for healing and achieving balance may help neutralize the stress we created."[23]

DO: Paint! Taking a painting or drawing class is a great way to learn how to observe without judging, especially the colors around you and the beauty in everyday things. The purpose of really seeing is to challenge that part of your programming that makes assumptions and jumps to conclusions. Once you stop thinking you know and begin observing, your mental chatter will start to dial down.

MOVE: Qi gong has many forms, some of which can be done seated. This ancient meditation practice is more of a moving meditation, good for the restless or sleepy. The gentle movements can keep you awake so you can take the rest of energy to turn it inward to enhance your meditation. Two DVD's I particularly like are *Qi Gong for Beginners* by Lee Holden and *Qi Gong* by Ken Cohen.

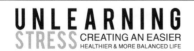

SUMMARY

Chapter 3: Be Seated

- Meditation and mindfulness provides the opportunity to see ourselves more clearly.

- Without inner-knowing, it is difficult to transform and heal.

- There are lots of meditation and mindfulness practices. These practices will help you to identify, harness, and transform your energy to maximize your healing.

- Build these techniques into your life so that your day to day life becomes your meditation.

FOOD FOR THOUGHT FOR CHAPTER 3

Where does your mind go when you try to be seated? Does it go to a threat? Is it worth your energy? If not, then why do you keep going there? Can you imagine that energy drain no longer occupying your energy? What will it take? Are you prepared to do whatever it takes to reclaim your mind and the present moment?

Did you try to meditate the 'right' way? Do you spend a lot of time trying to be 'right'?

If you were uncomfortable, what did you do? Did you change positions? Did you complain? Did you do something else? How does this reaction to being uncomfortable show up in other places in your life?

Did you experience a moment without being concerned with the past or the future?

What was your intention when you sat down to meditate? To be present? To be free? To be open? Can you carry out that intention throughout your day? Can you bring that intention to every moment of your life?

Chapter # 4 : Be Nourished

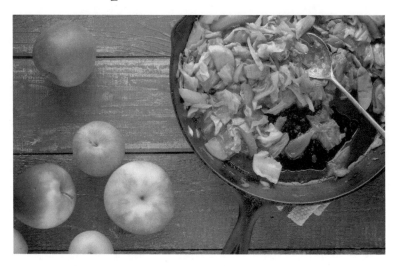

"I live on good soup, not on fine words"

— Moliere

When we dine together, we bond. "The story of the meal was a story of social relations and the notions of 'culture', that key attribute that we humans have, and other species lack,"[24] explains University Cambridge archeologist Martin Jones, author of *Feast: Why Humans Share Food*. The hearth has long nourished, comforted and helped us to connect – with each other and our own creativity.

But beware! What you ingest around this hearth is what you will become. I can't emphasize enough what an impact the food you eat has on your overall well-being. You are what you eat. Literally.

"What you put on your fork is the most powerful medicine you can take to correct the root causes of chronic disease," says Mark Hyman, MD, author of *The Blood Sugar Solution*.[25] Your diet contributes to autoimmune disorders, blood sugar issues and hormonal imbalances. The health of your thyroid, chronic fatigue, fibromyalgia, multiple sclerosis, neurological issues such as Parkinson's and Alzheimer's are also impacted. Your heart, blood pressure, and your susceptibility to cancer are also connected with diet. We can go on to include everything down to how you perform at any sports, managing your weight, and of course, managing your stress.

UNLEARNING STRESS CREATING AN EASIER HEALTHIER & MORE BALANCED LIFE

JAMES ROHR, L.Ac

We eat when we're happy. We eat when we're overwhelmed. We can use food to help us celebrate or to cope. We can try to eat our way out of depression or eat our way into our self-sabotage temporary comforts. Regardless of why you are eating, the food you eat has the power to turn your genes on or shut them off; it "speaks" to your genes.[26]

Our genes themselves haven't changed that much over time. Inside, you're still a cave (wo)man, but your environment has changed. Dramatically. Environmental changes alter how the genes behave or "express". It's becoming increasingly clear from the western perspective that most of our modern diseases, including obesity and metabolic syndrome, come from our genetics being out of synch with our environment (aka our food).[27] In fact, I think this disharmony between our bodily needs and our environment toxins is becoming the biggest stress threat these days. It is hard to be at peace when your body is fighting like hell to detoxify and eliminate toxins from the foods we've eaten.

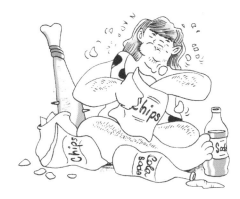

What many of us are eating these days, a mess of processed and packaged sugars, fake and unstable fats and just for good measure, heaps of salt, is the 'environment' that is killing us. While we love the taste (there's a reason no one can eat just one), these highly-processed foods don't love us back.

"The ultimate basis for most diet-related diseases results from the evolutionary discordance between our ancient and conservative genome and recently introduced foods," points out Dr. Loren Cordain, a pioneer on the paleo movement.[28] From mouthfuls of cavities to weaker bones to heart disease and autoimmune conditions galore, many (if not all) prevalent modern diseases can be traced back to eating foods that are harmful to your particular constitution. Instead of eating for health, we're eating our collective way to a fast and chemically-induced death.

TREAT DIGESTION FIRST

One of the primary books in Chinese medicine was written by Li Dong Yuan over 800 years ago. Entitled *Treatise on the Spleen and Stomach*, the book espouses the importance of ensuring a healthy digestion. This school of thought says that optimal health begins with a highly functioning digestive tract; poor digestion leads to poor overall health.

We think it is time to return to this method of treatment since so many millions of us lack healthy digestion. In the US alone, close to 65 million people suffer from chronic constipation[29] or have a specific digestive disorder, including:[30]

> 600,000 have Crohn's Disease: an autoimmune disorder (when your immune system malfunctions and attacks and destroys healthy tissue) and inflammatory bowel disease in which the body over-reacts and the gastrointestinal tract – the small intestine, large intestine, rectum and even the mouth – has chronic inflammation.[31]
>
> 1,000,000 – Ulcerative Colitis: an inflammatory bowel disease that affects the lining of the colon (the large intestine) and the rectum.[32] Basically, the colon has any number of open sores (ulcers) which cause a lot of abdominal pain and produce bloody diarrhea.[33]
>
> 3,000,000 - Celiac Disease: the lining of the small intestine becomes damaged and unable to absorb nutrients from food, which can lead to severe malnutrition. Interestingly, it can develop at any point in life, including late adulthood.[34]
>
> 60 Million – Irritable Bowel Syndrome (IBS) Unlike irritable bowel disease (like Crohn's and ulcerative colitis), the structure of the bowel isn't abnormal, but the sufferer still has abnormal pain and cramping, changes in bowel movement and swings between constipation and diarrhea. IBS can occur at any age, but most often starts in early adulthood and is twice as common in women.[35]

That's a lot of digestive distress. Even if you don't suffer from a diagnosed illness, you may still be sensitive to your food. Maybe you're extra bloated or gassy, maybe you get tired after you eat, or maybe you have chronic sinus issues. In many people, these symptoms can be traced back to diet.

BE NOURISHED

If you look hard enough, you can find advocates for just about every kind of diet you could dream up. I don't believe in any one specific diet for everyone; rather, use your body as a laboratory. Experiment with your food and stay vigilant about how you feel. Find the nutritional path that best suits you. In Chinese medicine, we recognize that each individual is unique. Your body gives you feedback all the time about your food and lifestyle choices. Learn to listen to it, make changes when necessary, and you'll start feeling better than ever before.

Whether you're getting your information from vegans, vegetarians, Hippocrates institute, Weston A. Price, nutrition.gov, South Beach, Paleo, Atkins, or anything else, it is up to you to find the diet that best suits your needs. And your needs may change over time! We have come across people who do well on a certain diet in the short term, but for a prolonged period of time, that diet can be detrimental. A juice fast may be great for a week because you've stopped eating the junk food that was doing so much harm. But over time, you won't get all the nutrients you need just from maple syrup and lemons. The key, as with most things, is balance.

Focus on organic, humanely and locally grown food. Amish and local small farmers can be a great resource.

With love and respect to all different nutritional schools of thought, here are some guidelines we suggest following when it comes to what you put into your mouth:

EAT REAL FOOD

Preferably organic, humanely and locally grown. Avoid those nasty genetically modified organisms (GMO). If you can get your foods from a local farmers market or co-op for organic local produce that is great. If you eat meat and dairy, get it form a healthy farm source, as in an Amish farm or close-by farming community. Do what you can to know where your food comes from. The cleaner the food, the less involved your immune system will be. The more your immune system can rest, the more energy you'll have to be playful.

Remember the last time you cut yourself? Your wound became inflamed, puffy and tender to the touch. The swelling, redness and pain of inflammation is how your body isolates invading germs and toxins and deactivates them; under the right circumstances, inflammation is how you start to heal and how the rest of your body is protected from the infected wound site. This is a healthy response to a temporary problem.

Now imagine that same response happening throughout the many feet of digestive tract that you have. Your body may be responding to bacteria, viruses, or any other "foreigners" your body doesn't like or can't recognize, such as over-processed, chemically and genetically modified food.

It's bad enough that we're eating nutritionally-devoid crap, but we continue to assault our poor bodies with it day after day, week after week, year after year. And our immune systems never get a much-needed day off because it's so busy constantly dealing with the continuous smoldering fire of inflammation in your vital organs and other important innards. This opens the door to heart disease, cancer, diabetes, dementia and all manner of chronic diseases.[36]

If we are eating 'dead' food, then we aren't getting adequate nutritional support we need to heal. "People who eat toxic, nutrient-poor diets are more likely to contract chronic infections and do not easily recover from them," note Paul and Shou-Ching Shih Jaminet – respectively a Ph.D. in astrophysics and a Ph.D. in molecular biology (and a cancer researcher at Beth Israel Deaconess Medical Center and Harvard Medical School) and co-authors of *Perfect Health Diet: Four Steps to Renewed Health, Youthful Vitality and Long Life*. "Disease, premature aging, and impaired health have 3 primary causes: food toxicity, malnutrition, and chronic infections...These 3 causes go together."[37]

EAT A VARIETY

Let's include meat, fish, veggies, tubers, and some fruit into the 'prioritize these' list. While any food can create issues for any particular individual, in broad strokes, these are typically nutrient-dense and not too abrasive or irritating to the body. "Lean proteins [from wild-caught fish and cattle grazed exclusively on grasses] support strong muscles, healthy bones and optimal immune function," advises Robb Wolf, author of *The Paleo Solution*. "Fruits and vegetables are rich in antioxidants, vitamins, minerals and phytonutrients that have been shown to decrease the likelihood of developing a number of degenerative diseases including cancer, diabetes and neurological decline."[38]

EAT SEASONALLY

Nowadays we can import fruits and veggies from around the world. We've lost touch with what is 'in season' and what is not. As mentioned in the introduction, a watermelon in winter time is contrary to the natural flow of things. If you focus on eating seasonally, then you are eating foods that are grown/sprouted/hatched/flowering instead of foods made in a laboratory somewhere. Your ecological footprint is less and according to Chinese medicine, the tastes and flavors of the foods will most likely balance out the environmental dangers of that particular season. That is, foods that are more prevalent in the summertime tend to clear away internal heat while foods and spices that crop up in the fall and winter tend to be more warming to help fight off that internal chill. As we've said all along so far, health has a lot to do with your interaction with all facets of your environment. Shop at your local farmer's market or co-op, and eat with the seasons to re-immerse yourself into a cycle that has less resistance.

CHEW YOUR FOOD

Digestion starts in your mouth. Take your time, practice those deep breaths, chew and enjoy your food. The more your chew your food, the easier it is for your body to assimilate the nutrients. Slow down and savor the flavor of what you're eating. This alone can be enough to get you to start eating better food. When we actually take the time to be present and mindful of the flavors of what we are eating, then we may not want to satiate ourselves with salt upon fat upon salt upon fat. We may actually start craving a variety of textures and spices. Try putting your fork down between bites or chewing your food twenty to fifty times before swallowing. Your jaw will get a workout and your stomach will thank you.

EAT (HEALTHY) FATS AND OILS

To function, your body and brain both need fuel. Like an engine, the better suited the fuel is, the better you will function. If you are designed to run on regular gasoline and you put diesel in the tank (and vice versa), eventually there will be problems. In biological terms, this means providing your body with fuel that requires little or no energy to convert and leaves few to none toxic byproducts when burned. When your body stores energy from food to use later, it stores it mostly as a fatty acid of the "long-chain" sort – the ones that remain solid at room temperature (like butter) – and you! Fats are useful to balance your mood, improve energy, and actually to help control your weight.

BUT WHAT ABOUT MY CHOLESTEROL? Cholesterol is a waxy substance so important to your health that every cell in your body can manufacture it. The lion's share of your cholesterol is used by the brain. So every cell can make cholesterol and the brain needs most of it. Think cholesterol is important?

Cholesterol is one of the prime building materials for memory; when you sleep, your body manufactures it in order to help neurons communicate. Interfere with this communication, say by artificially lowering your cholesterol, and people start to have trouble forming new memories and act like they're in the early stages of Alzheimer's. This is why people taking cholesterol-lowering drugs, called statins - the #1 selling category of pharmaceuticals prescribed - often complain of memory loss. Statins artificially lower your cholesterol levels, but at quite the cost.

In addition to making memories, cholesterol acts as a kind of an internal "Band-Aid". When your arteries tear microscopically, cholesterol is brought to the scene of the injury to smooth over the cracks and let the lining heal. Think of Emergency Medical Techs and paramedics showing up at the scene of an accident to attend to the immediate damage. What the EMTs didn't do was cause the accident; they merely showed up in response. And the bigger the accident, the more EMTs. Just as holding the EMTs responsible for the accident makes no sense, similarly, cholesterol is a first-responder, not a causal factor.

What typically is a causal factor of tears in arteries is inflammation. Inflammation that is often caused by a diet high in too much refined sugar, fake trans fats and eating stuff that does a number on your blood sugar. So unless you inherited hypercholesterolemia, instead of attacking the peacemaker, go after a big cause of trouble: eating the wrong stuff. Your big, cholesterol-fueled brain thanks you.

MORE ON OILS

Beware of 'vegetable oils'. They line supermarket shelves, prominently proclaiming how "heart healthy" they are - sunflower oil, safflower oil, corn oil, canola oil, soybean oil. Soybean oil, in particular, is present in so much of the processed food we eat that in the US alone, it accounts for 20% of people's daily calories. This is a huge upheaval in the way we eat, dating back as recently as the industrial revolution when the technology came about which enabled businesses to extract the oil from these crops and start marketing them as veggie oils.

"The term 'vegetable oil' has come to encompass all those yellowy looking oils, and an ingredient of almost every product you find, on the inside shelves of a grocery store," explains Penny McIntosh, certified personal trainer, nutritional counselor and health coach. "A more accurate term is 'industrial seed oil'…a petroleum produced, overheated, oxidized and chemically-deodorized, man-man product that is made from seeds that are genetically modified and full of pesticides and we have been led to believe are healthy."[39]

Oils that we recommend cooking with are butter, tallow and lard (yes, we like it the old fashioned way). Coconut oil and grapeseed oil can also be ok, but as a general rule, be very careful with any non-butter or lard cooking at high temperatures. Oils such as olive oil, sesame or flax oil we don't recommend heating at all; rather, use them cold or room temperature as a salad dressing.

EAT FERMENTED

It's not that bacteria and viruses are new, but the weapons in our health arsenal are in short supply these days. We now eat so much less of the foods that once provided us with plentiful amounts of gut-friendly, 'good' bacteria: traditionally fermented fare. The main way that food was preserved in ye olden days before refrigeration was lacto-fermentation. From sauerkraut to kimchi to other pickled veggies, these are replete with probiotics which supported our natural immune response against diseases, viruses and pathogens.

Now that most of us no longer eat traditionally-fermented foods, our immunity has paid the price. "Scientists and doctors today are mystified by the proliferation of new viruses--not only the deadly AIDS virus but the whole gamut of human viruses that seem to be associated with everything from chronic fatigue to cancer and arthritis," explain Sally Fallon and Mary Enig, PhD, authors of Know Your Fats. "They are equally mystified by recent increases in the incidence of intestinal parasites and pathogenic yeasts, even among those whose sanitary practices are faultless. Could it be that in abandoning the ancient practice of lacto-fermentation and in our insistence on a diet in which everything has been pasteurized, we have compromised the health of our intestinal flora and made ourselves vulnerable to legions of pathogenic microorganisms?"[40]

Your gut contains over 500 different species of bacteria weighing a good three pounds, housing a teeming population of trillions of microbial cells. "Think of your gut as one big ecosystem," advises Dr. Hyman. An ecosystem which controls everything from digestion, to metabolism, inflammation and cancer risk – and even various vitamins and nutrients. But eat too much processed food and it actually weeds out much of the bacterial variety, concentrating what's left in a way that's unhealthy.

When we eat generic, sterilized food, we reduce the jungle in our guts and our protection against disease.

When researchers recently compared the gut bacteria of children eating a high-fiber diet in Burkina Faso with Italian children in Florence eating a more Western diet – double the calories and half the fiber – they discovered that the African kids' micro biomes were dominated by a group of bacteria which specialize in breaking down plant fibers, the Bacteroidetes, while the Italian kids bowels had a lot of bacteria seen in obese people, the Fimicutes.

When we eat generic, sterilized food, we reduce the jungle in our guts and our protection against disease. "An unbalanced or simplified micro biome could be *damaging the health of Westerners more directly*, affecting the risk of a variety of other medical conditions, including allergies, inflammatory bowel disease, bowel cancer and *obesity*," opined the researcher. "A diverse micro biome could also prevent more harmful species from setting up shop – indeed, and somewhat unexpectedly, food poisoning bacteria like Shigella and Escherichia were less common in the Burkinabe children than the Italian ones."[41]

Protect your micro biome by feeding it the good bacteria it loves. Before refrigeration, people stored perishable foods by using fermentation. Roman soldiers fueled their takeover of the known world on fermented bread – a sourdough, which literally comes from a starter-dough that's fermented sour. One of Korea's most famous foods is the pungent fermented cabbage dish kimchi. Central Asians pride themselves on their fermented mare's milk, kumis, Ethiopians on their injera bread, San Franciscans on their sour dough (Le Pain Quotidian and Trader Joe's are both good brands)[42], while the French sure do love their crème fraiche.

In addition to preserving a food, fermenting it makes nutrition it contains much more accessible and is capable of completely transforming an otherwise inedible food, such as grains. "Grain fermentation is widespread in Africa and is probably nearly as old as agriculture on the continent," explains Dr. Guyenet. Like the West African porridge Ogi that is a staple in the region. The whole grain - millet, sorghum or corn – is first soaked for up to three days, then mixed with water in order to remove some of the tough outer layer (the bran – which they feed to their livestock). What's left over from being wet-milled is then fermented for another two to three days, after which, a week has elapsed and it's finally cooked into an edible porridge. "The nutritional importance of fermentation is suggested by the amount of time and effort that many African cultures put into it," adds Guyenet, "when they could save themselves a lot of trouble by simply soaking and cooking their grains."[43]

GRASS FED, ORGANS, AND EGGS

If you're going to eat meat, make sure it is grass fed. Why? Grass fed meat, aka meat from animals grazed entirely on grass, such as cows, sheep, and bison, are fantastic sources of protein. However, be aware that the meat from animals raised in a commercial Concentrated Animal Feeding Operation (CAFO) has a much different fatty acid profile than grass-fed, in particular, because instead of eating grass, for the latter part of its life, CAFO cattle is fed grain, which it is allergic to, requiring vast quantities of antibiotics so its feed doesn't kill it. Plus the grain feed makes the fatty acids in the meat more inflammatory. CAFO cows are brought to the full slaughter weight faster thanks to hormones. And yes, all this stuff ends up in the meat. Cows raised ethically and slaughtered humanely are healthier and produce far-superior, nutrient-rich meat. If you must buy CAFO meat, opt for leaner cuts to cut back on the potential for toxins.

When grandma had that weekly liver and onions, she knew what she was doing nutritionally. From calcium to magnesium, to Vitamins A through E to the important Bs, 100g of liver (a little over 3 ounces) trounces veggie "superfoods" including apples and carrots by factors of 2 to 100. An argument against eating an animal's liver is that it's where toxins are stored, however, this isn't quite true. In fact, the liver is more of a toxin transit-station: it neutralizes poisons, chemicals and drugs but then sends them on to the fat tissue to be stored there. What the liver does actually store are Vitamins A, D, E, K, folic acid, B12, copper and iron. Again, as with regular cuts of meat, buying organ meats from animals grown and raised on pasture is the far superior choice for your nutritional buck. Other organ meats to consider adding to your menu, or stewed in the Crock Pot with lots of veggies and aromatic "ick-factor-disguising" spices, include kidney, tongue, heart, brains (sweetbreads) and trips.

Don't be afraid of pastured eggs, yolk and all! The egg may have been the original superfood. Properly pastured eggs are laid by chickens allowed to live with dignity and spend their days engaged in chicken'y activities – enjoying the fresh air and sunshine, scratching in the dirt, pecking at seeds and insects and moving about getting exercise. And compared to the eggs laid by chickens packed into vast sheds and raised on feed toxic enough that you have to wear protective gear to be around it, the pastured eggs are like a different species of egg altogether. When Mother Earth News tested them, they found that where conventional eggs contained an average of 487 IU of Vitamin A, pastured eggs had almost double the Vitamin A; Vitamin D levels were an astounding 136-204IU compared with conventional's 34IU; and vitamin E, Beta-carotene and Omega 3 fatty acids were similarly more loaded in the pastured eggs.[44]

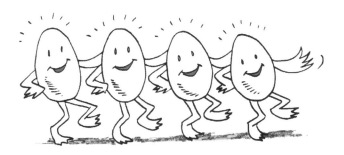

The yolk contains 100% of certain compounds, called carotenoids, which are concentrated in the back of the eye and are thought to protect against age-related loss of sight, along with essential fatty acids, vitamins A, E, D and K. The yolk, like its golden hue, is nutritional gold and also rich in calcium, iron, phosphorus, zinc, thiamin, B6, folate, B12 and pantothenic acid, as well as copper, manganese and selenium. And the whites? Other than protein, not much. "The only thing that could justify their consumption is their attachment to their companion yolk," says cholesterol expert Chris Masterjohn, PhD. "In fact, the slew of nutrients in an egg yolk is so comprehensive," he adds, "that a few a eggs would offer better insurance than a multi-vitamin."[45] From all-too-common deficiencies in magnesium, calcium, folate and vitamins A, E, B6 and copper, eating egg yolks regularly is a simple way to solve most of your common nutritional deficiencies.

THE HIDDEN TOXINS

What do diabetes, heart disease, autoimmune disorders – including Multiple Sclerosis, Rheumatoid Arthritis, Lupus and Vitiligo – Alzheimer's, osteoporosis and obesity have in common? They didn't exist in almost the entirety of our 2.5 million year history as humans – until maybe 10,000 or so years ago. What happened? Diet changes, primarily. "Diet is one of the major determinants of chronic-disease risk," agrees Guyenet.[46] We started eating foods at odds with our health, starting with the fruits of agriculture, namely

- grains
- industrial seed cooking oils made from corn, safflower, soybean, or cottonseed
- sugar (especially high fructose corn syrup)
- soy in all its myriad forms (milk, flour, protein)

The reason to watch out for these four nutritional demons is they do one (or all) of a few bad things to your health. They mess with your nutritional status, digestive comfort, and/or your insides in general, causing internal inflammation. This inflammation is thought to lay the groundwork for just about every other modern disease.

> *Technically, whole grains are loaded with lots of excellent vitamin and minerals. Unfortunately, they are not in a form that our bodies can access and use easily.*

GO AGAINST THE GRAIN

WHOLE GRAINS= LEAKY GUTS Whole grains, especially wheat, are praised as "heart healthy" and enjoy an awesome reputation… that is completely undeserved, primarily because they contain the protein gluten – found in wheat, barley, rye, spelt and oats. When eaten, especially in excess, gluten damages the lining of the intestine, allowing undigested particles of food and other forms of digestive nastiness to escape back into the body, making the gut "leaky" and sending the immune system into a tizzy. Once the body detects these foreign particles, the immune system begins to attack itself. Translation: you don't feel good.

PHARAOH'S CURSE The relatively new (in evolutionary terms) grain-based diet cultivated by the Ancient Egyptians did a number on their health. They seemed to have primarily a 'heart healthy lifestyle' being active, eating lots of veggies and fruit, not smoking, eating only a small amount of meat and not yet inventing junk food, fake trans-fats, or high fructose corn syrup. However, they frequently ate honey-sweetened cakes and lots of bread. When mummies dating from as early as 1500 B.C.E. were examined via CT scan, the majority had major hardening of their arteries at age 40. "We were a bit surprised, adds a radiologist on the research team, "by just how much atherosclerosis we found on ancient Egyptians who were young."[47]

They didn't eat the junk food we do, they ate a lot of breads and other grain-based dishes. And their clogged arteries gave them heart disease and killed them. "Commonly, we think of coronary artery or heart disease as a consequence of our modern lifestyles," notes Dr. Gregory Thomas, a clinical professor of cardiology at UC Irvine who lead a research team studying CT scans of ancient Egyptian royalty. "Our results point to a missing link in our understanding of heart disease, because if this were the case, why would ancient Egyptians with lifestyles so different from ours have atherosclerosis?"[48]

BUT IT'S HEART-HEALTHY! Technically, yes, whole grains are loaded with lots of excellent vitamin and minerals. Unfortunately, they are not in a form that our bodies can access and use easily. Many of the commonly-accepted measures of how nutritious a food is - such as the ANDI score or Joel Fuhrman's Nutrient Density scale - are based on the nutrition contained in the foods before they are cooked. The reason the term "before they are cooked" matters is that when foods are cooked or otherwise processed for consumption (eg. sprouting or fermenting), it changes how much nutrition is available for your body to access and use, aka its bioavailability.

Bioavailability is the key and is what matters most when it comes to how nutritious a food is. Instead of practicing nutrition in a vacuum, what makes a lot more sense is to look at how bioavailable a particular food's nutrient density is when we eat it. Items such as whole grains, wheat and legumes in their unaltered state rate well in terms of their nutrient density. However, when cooked, they are completely unimpressive.

"I believe that a combination of chronic stress, genetic vulnerability, nutrient deficiencies and food toxins (including gluten) are responsible for most of the chronic disease in the western world, including mental illness," opined Emily Deans, MD – a practicing psychiatrist in Massachusetts – in *Psychology Today*. Consuming wheat and possibly even pasteurized dairy is increasingly being linked to everything from schizophrenia, bipolar disorder, autism thanks to possible neuroactive peptides from "milk and grain products ...that can enter into the circulation and ultimately cross the blood-brain barrier."[49] Yike*s*.

BEWARE SUGAR AND HIGH-FRUCTOSE CORN SYRUP

Researchers confirmed in a study of the impact of eating junk food on depression. "The more fast food you consume, the greater the risk of depression," notes the lead author of the study. "Even eating small quantities is linked to a significantly higher chance of developing depression." [50]

Sugar, sugar everywhere! The white stuff, and the better-living-thru-chemistry stuff, high-fructose corn syrup, is in salad dressings, marinades, candy bars, processed foods, sodas and more. Often, there is so much sugar added to a product that the manufacturer will list the sugar-added by specific type because just calling it sugar means it would end up as the first ingredient listed. When you're playing label detective, the easiest way to spot sugar in its many guises is the ending –ose, as in: glucose, fructose, sucrose, dextrose, maltose, lactose, levulose. The other ending to be on the lookout for is –tol: mannitol, and sorbitol.[51]

We know that you know sugar is not good for you or your health, but allow us to reiterate. Refined sugar can impair how your white blood cells function, which impairs your immune system, it "switches off" a key hormone which tells you you're full (called leptin), it can make you more "resistant" to insulin, precipitating Type II diabetes – and the witch's brew of health troubles that brings and might very well "feed" cancer cells.[52] "Sugar-sweetened beverages are probably one of the most fattening elements of the modern diet," adds Guyenet. "Sugar can be fattening in certain contexts, specifically if it is added to foods and beverages to increase their palatability, reward value and energy density."[53]

Suffice it to say that for maximum glowing health and peace of mind, you don't want sugar on the brain. "Sugar is almost identical to alcohol biochemically," observes clinical psychologist Julia Ross, M.A., author of *The Diet Cure* and the executive director of Recovery Systems, a California clinic specializing in treating addictions and disorders of mood and eating. "Both sugar and alcohol instantly skyrocket blood sugar levels and temporarily raise levels of at least two potent mood chemicals in the brain."[54]

JUNK FOOD

When you eat something, your taste buds send signals to parts of the brain which control your breathing, digestion and other involuntary processes, which then activate the cells containing the molecules which respond to pleasure, the endorphins or opioids. "Whether the opioid circuits are activated by highly palatable foods or by drugs," explains David Kessler, MD, the former FDA commissioner and author of *The End of Overeating*, "they enable the body to perceive a rewarding experience."[55] In particular, when you combine sugar, fat and salt in specific combinations, you can generate behavior on the part of people that borders on addiction. The palatability of food doesn't just mean it "tastes good", it also measures the degree to which it stimulates your appetite, both before eating and when you decide you want to stop.

"Palatability does involve taste, of course, but, crucially, it also involves the motivation to pursue that taste," adds Kessler. "And it's that stimulation, or the anticipation of that stimulation, rather than genuine hunger, that makes us put food into our mouths long after our caloric needs are satisfied."[56] Most of what you buy at fast food joints or eat in chain restaurants isn't "home cooked" or "fresh", rather it's designed by food chemists to be so palatable as to change your neural circuitry and "encode" it so you develop a strong taste for it. In other words, it messes with your brain, and your control over your actions.

The point of this is not to revive scary memories of high school biology class; rather it's to point out that what you eat can directly impact – and even alter – the brain's pathways. Eating foods that create addictive behaviors do little or nothing for long-term peace of mind.. Or, to put it a little differently: soul searching is hard when you're fixating on your next fix.

ONLY FERMENTED SOY

The foods made from soy eaten in Asia traditionally have two very specific qualities that differentiate them from the ubiquitous soy-in-everything in the west. They fermented the soy into items like natto, miso and tamari in order to neutralize the potent toxins. Unfermented soy can be harmful to the pancreas and thyroid, and it can impact estrogen levels, encouraging certain types of tumors to grow. I suggest avoiding soy products that have been processed and haven't been fermented, including soy milk, tofu, soy protein isolate, flour, and, of course, soybean oil.

SO NOW WHAT?!

Use your body as a laboratory. Elimination diets are a good way to begin to identify the foods that are causing you the most harm. Pick something that you eat often and that you suspect is causing a problem and eliminate it. Notice how you feel. In some cases, people may notice dramatic improvements after just a couple of days of elimination. Other times, you may need to eliminate it for a month or two. When you want to reintroduce a certain food, add it in once and wait five days. If your symptoms haven't returned, try again a few days apart. If no symptoms appear, then this food should now be 'safe' for your constitution. Continue this process of elimination and addition until you have come up with a diet that isn't aggravating to your system.

> ### BUT WHAT ABOUT SOY SAUCE?
>
> *It not only contains soy, but wheat as well. A double no-no. Instead, try Coconut Aminos. Taste-wise, it's a dead-ringer for soy sauce, but in addition to tasting great, it's also loaded with aminos, vitamins and minerals.*

You may still need more variety, and possibly supplementation, to get your body all the nutrients it needs. But, if you are very symptomatic, controlling the initial inflammation is important, and an elimination diet can be very helpful. Clinically, we see that eliminating dairy, gluten, and yeast are the biggest culprits.

Looking for a more precise approach? There is a relatively new group of labs that are popping up where they test for IGG reactions. These are a slower allergic response that the body is mounting, in this case, to the food that we eat. These are not the peanut allergy that makes your throat close. Rather, these IGG reactions manifest more commonly as frequent bloating, constipation, diarrhea, sinus congestion, inflammation/pain, fatigue, depression, and more. When we eat too much of these foods, the body is wasting valuable energy fighting the allergen. This triggers a whole bunch of not-so-fun-feeling symptoms. Amazingly, when these foods are removed from someone's diet, symptoms often disappear within a couple of days. The key is to find out what foods your body loves and which ones it struggles with.

ADD SOME SPICE

One of the best sources of the fat-soluble vitamins that support your immune system, including Vitamin A, is high-vitamin cod liver oil, in particular, fermented CLO. "Fermenting the livers of fish to extract the oil is an old world practice that may go back as far as biblical times," points out Dave Wetzel of Green Pasture, which produces the gold-standard in pristine fermented CLO from wild-caught fish. Their *BLUE ICE line of fermented CLO blended with high-vitamin Butter Oil* (if you're squeamish, opt for the capsules) the "X Factor" identified by Dr. Weston A. Price in fighting tooth decay is one of the best ways to get your Vitamin A, D and K.

PILL IT: If you're a just-in-case type, then you might want to add some probiotics to your daily regimen. Nebraska Cultures specializes in high-quality blends of probiotic microorganisms that include L. acidophilus DDS-1 to protect against gas, bloating and diarrhea. They market it under the label *Dr. Shahani's*.

EAT IT: Add some sauerkraut or kimchi to your day. It's easy to make and enjoy with meals as a quick source of healthy probiotics. Alternatively, if you have a hankering to make your own fermented veggies, the godfather of all things fermented is undoubtedly Sandor Katz. He authored *Wild Fermentation*, which contains over 100 recipes from a wide range of traditions, including Cherokee, African, Japanese and Russian. "Many of your favorite foods and drinks are probably fermented," says Katz, citing as examples: bread, cheese, wine, beer, cider, mead, pickles, kraut, kimchi, chocolate, coffee, tea, salami, miso, tempeh, soy sauce, vinegar, kefir and of course, kraut.[57]

DRINK IT: An easy way to scarf down 1 billion or so probiotics while getting your refreshment on is with the fizzy fermented (but non-alcoholic) tea, Kombucha. Alternatively, kefir, a liquid yogurt-like bevy is also loaded with probiotics.

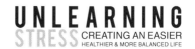

READ: The key vitamins most of us are deficient in can be found in foods for the most part, with a few exceptions. We recommend following up with *Perfect Health Diet: Four Steps to Renewed Health, Youthful Vitality and Long Life,*[58] and *The Blood Sugar Solution* by Mark Hyman, MD for more details.

GET TESTED: Check out Immunolabs for their IGG testing and to find a doctor nearby who can get it ordered for you.

WATCH: short but sweet TEDx videos - *"Minding Your Mitchondria"* (how real food almost completely reversed one woman's multiple sclerosis) *The American Diet* (learn the complete history of how the food we eat changed in the last 150 years in under 20 minutes!)

PREPARE: a feel-good feast and enjoy with people you care about with seasonal, traditional dishes featured in a *Full Moon Feast: Food and the Hunger for Connection* by Jessica Prentice. Be sure to treat your ears to a feast while you prepare one by downloading something fun like *COOKING MUSIC: Ivory Coast, Ghana, Senegal and Ecuador.*

READ: *Fat: an Appreciation of a Misunderstood Ingredient* (with Recipes); *Eat with Your Hands* by chef Zak Pelaccio; *Savor: Mindful Eating, Mindful Life* by Thich Nhat Hanh; *Nourishing Traditions: The Cookbook that Challenges Politically Correct Nutrition; Nutrition and Physical Degeneration* by Dr. Weston A. Price; *The Paleo Solution: The Original Human Diet* by Robb Wolf; *Practical Paleo: A Customized Approach to Health and a Whole Foods Lifestyle* by Diane Sanfilippo; *Healing with Whole Foods* by Paul Pitchford; and *The Cholesterol Myth* by Dr. Jonny Bowden and Dr. Steven Sinatra

TRY: A new and possibly "scary" food (such as traditional sheep's head, fermented mare's milk, or seagull). A pair of food-obsessed researchers in Norway found that eating food you found frightening is as exciting as adventure tourism.[59]

UNLEARNING
STRESS CREATING AN EASIER
HEALTHIER & MORE BALANCED LIFE

SUMMARY

Chapter 4: Be Nourished

- Without adequate nutrition, there is a limit to how healthy a body can be.

- Many diseases facing the modern population are in some way related to improper nutrition.

- Fat is no longer a bad word. Be sure to get adequate amounts of healthy fats so your body has what it needs to feel better.

- No matter which diet you choose, use your body as a laboratory. Keep a food journal, writing down everything you eat and how you feel physically, mentally, and emotionally. After a week or two, review your journal and look for correlations between what you've eaten and any bloating, fatigue, anxiety, panic attacks, and/or pain, etc.

FOOD FOR THOUGHT FOR CHAPTER 4

What resistance are you finding towards making dietary changes?

Are you having cravings?

Are you stuck with habits?

Are you a creature of comfort?

If you didn't have that craving, how would your life be different? Can you imagine a week without this craving? What would you eat or do instead?

What is one dietary change you can make today and follow it all day?

What is one food you can eliminate today that you know does not do well in your body?

What is one food you can eat today that will help you feel better?

Did you notice a connection between your stress tolerance/patience and what you ate today?

Chapter # 5 : Be Grateful

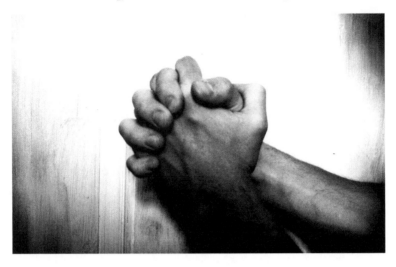

Bless, O Lord, this food we are about to eat; and we pray You, O God, that it may be good for our body and soul; and if there be any poor creature hungry or thirsty walking along the road, send them into us that we can share the food with them, just as You share your gifts with all of us.

— Irish Prayer for Grace

An easy way to practice counting your blessings is to start with food. Food, as discussed at length in Chapter #4, is special in the way it nourishes on so many levels: body, mind, soul.

Before putting any goodness to your lips, take a moment to give thanks for such a tasty dish. This doesn't have to mean bowing your head and "saying grace". A simple internal acknowledgement that you're lucky enough to have something good to eat will suffice. This is not only good manners, but also helps to quiet down that pesky fight or flight response!

Saying thank you is like the "Open Sesame!" of fairy tales: those two little words contain power and magic.

When you say "thank you" and mean it, you defuse pathological energy and replace it with receptivity. This entirely changes your stress cycle. You are imbuing your environment with love and positivity while diluting any toxic

UNLEARNING STRESS CREATING AN EASIER HEALTHIER & MORE BALANCED LIFE

JAMES ROHR, L.Ac

experiences. This will help activate that PNS, which, as you may remember from Chapter #2, allows your body to repair and heal.

But don't think you have to save up your gratitude for something big. The gratitude can be for something really impressive, like a great promotion, or something more ordinary, like taking a deep breath, or something tricky, like the illness you're suffering from. Yes, I just suggested being thankful for your illness. Stay with me and I'll explain why.

"If the only prayer you ever said in your whole life was 'thank you,' noted the 13th century German theologian and philosopher Meister Eckhart, "that would suffice."

Being grateful has been shown to be more than a whole lot of wishful-thinking. One study had people train some of their character "strengths", including gratitude. After 10 weeks, the subjects demonstrated a significant increase in wellbeing, cheerfulness and feeling satisfied with life.[60] Another study found that teens that were grateful were more likely to be happy and less likely to have behavior problems at school or abuse drugs and alcohol. Overall, the grateful teens had a much better sense of well-being. When college students wrote letters every other week expressing gratitude, the majority found that their satisfaction with life soared, along with it their grades and their immune health.[61]

"These findings suggest that gratitude may be strongly linked with life-skills such as cooperation, purpose, creativity and persistence and, as such, gratitude is vital resource that parents, teachers and others who work with young people should help youth build as they grow up," noted the lead-researcher of the teen study. "More gratitude may be precisely what our society needs to raise a generation that is ready to make a difference in the world."[62] Being grateful is a like a megadose of insta-happiness,[63] a booster-shot in the arm of a romantic relationship[64] and even an assuager of power-abusing bosses. [65]

UNLEARNING
STRESS CREATING AN EASIER
HEALTHIER & MORE BALANCED LIFE

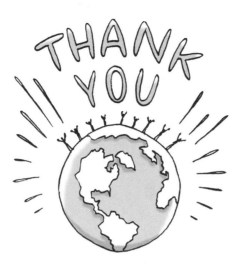

But if it's so simple to do and the results so powerful, then why are we so reluctant to be grateful?

Take getting sick, for example. From the physical symptoms to the way an illness can disrupt your life, getting sick is the opposite of fun. And when it happens, we usually react the way we always have: kneejerk-negative. And instead of looking at illness as an opportunity to re-examine our thoughts, feelings, and actions, we become angry. The feelings of disgust and frustration that happen after already being sick complicate the healing process by leading to more weakness and disease in the body. But your illness, just like every other roadblock in life, can become a stepping stone to your greatest moments.

BE GRATEFUL

To break out of the cycle of being a victim, of feeling like things are always being done to us, come from a place of accountability. I simply assume that everything I feel, think, interact with, and attract into life is a byproduct of my energy. Whether this is 'true' or not, by feeling like I have input into the events in my life, I realize I have the power to do something about them. We may not always be able to control everything that happens to us, but we can certainly control how we react to it.

UNLEARNING
STRESS CREATING AN EASIER
HEALTHIER & MORE BALANCED LIFE

JAMES ROHR, L.Ac

So when we say "thank you" for something, anything, we are honoring our life and our ability to create and manifest everything that makes us us. Even if what you're creating is illness – the "thank-you" is a way to start to eliminate some of that pathological energy you've been storing up. Being "thankful" for illness may seem ridiculous at first, but maybe this very absurdity may make you smile and start to undo the robotic programming that makes us react the same way every time. When we release ourselves from the confines of the same old behavior, same old reaction, and the same old story, we begin laying the groundwork for different, and usually much better, health.

Don't be overwhelmed at the notion of creating your calamities or illnesses. It is precisely that same power that can create illness that can also create healing. You're a creator of your life. I assume that illness doesn't appear out of nowhere and for no reason. While we may not always know the how or why, don't let this not knowing stop you from extracting the gifts illness can bring. Appreciate life and be grateful for all it entails.

(OVER)REACTIONS

The easiest way to get your head in the gratitude game is to practice what you learned in Chapter #3 and start observing your thoughts and reactions. Don't judge the reaction, just observe it. Avoiding getting sucked into the drama of the thought will help you to refocus on your goal of gratitude. Don't be afraid of the strong emotions that may arise, especially during a focused period of meditation.

The snow-globe is being jostled and our dormant emotions may start pouring down on us. But, remember, the hottest fires

Can't think of anything to be grateful for? The next time you feel the urge to go to the bathroom, hold it for as long as you can. (But don't do this often because holding it for too long too often can create problems.) Enjoy the sweet relief that comes from finally letting it flow. See? It is the little things that can make a huge difference.

remove the most impurities. When we become aware of the stories/dramas/ people/agencies that are making us the most upset, we see where we need to focus more of energy of gratitude and transformation.

We become aware of the choice we have to either stay pissed off/hurt/betrayed, or we can be thankful for the opportunity to breathe and be alive. In the beginning, both choices may seem difficult. Choose your hard. But, trust me, in the long run, gratitude pays much larger dividends.

UNMET EXPECTATIONS

When you expect something to happen, you do something unfortunate: you separate yourself from the "now". This is like taking an Express Train to the Ghetto of Unhappiness. You may have…

> … expected life to work out easily.
>
> … expected your birth parents to have kept you instead of giving you up for adoption.
>
> … expected a relative stranger, say, your doctor, to know precisely the words you wanted to hear and how you wanted to hear them.
>
> … expected the government to protect you from companies that poisoned the soil, triggering your autoimmune condition.

When a deep injury is done us, we never recover until we forgive.

Alan Paton,

South African Writer and

Educator (1903-1988)

Bring these unexamined or 'compartmentalized' thoughts to the foreground. Ask yourself why you have expectations of others. Because that's how it is in fairy tales? Because your friends never got sick so why did you? Because you believe there is a common decency that the world should adhere to? Shoulds and expectations keep you stuck in the past or obsessed about the future.

Your pointer finger may be locked and loaded to assign blame in all directions. But it is your stored resentments that will fester like a disgusting parasite, eating and consuming you even when you're not aware of it. **Unresolved blame stagnates the body's energy.** How can a pill, massage, acupuncture needle, or anything else provide long lasting relief without you relinquishing this resentment?

Instead of slinging blame and resentment everywhere, be grateful for things turning out differently. You hear stories of people who were sidetracked and avoided catastrophe. There are numerous stories of people who were supposed to be in the World Trade Center on 9/11 and for one reason or another, they weren't there that day. Maybe their car broke down, they were sick, missed a plane, or whatever. They could have been super pissed at the time that the world was not following their plan. And then, after catastrophe was averted, they realized they were granted a gift. Think of this any time you get delayed, absented or re-routed for whatever the reason. It might actually be saving you.

FORGIVENESS

Forgiveness is another approach to eliminate our toxic energy and create more room for gratitude. In order for gratitude to flourish, we have to forgive ourselves and those we feel have wronged us. As angry or upset as you may be, and as difficult as forgiveness may seem, the time has come to move your energy. Not sure who or what you may need to forgive? We hit on a few of them above with our unmet expectations, but let's take a closer look at some favorite objects of affection/obsession.

FORGIVE YOUR BODY

People tend to expect, or feel entitled, to a body that works perfectly (often without putting any extra effort into it). When our body malfunctions, the tendency is to get frustrated, look for blame, and/or feel like a victim. You may feel like your unspoken contract with the universe has been shattered once your body started to fail you. Why do you think that life was meant to be easy with a body that never faltered? Even if you've never had an issue up until recently, feeling betrayed doesn't help you to heal.

When we live hard, don't take care of ourselves, or interfere with the natural flow of energy with high stress and toxic relationships, individual cells are at a higher risk for being compromised.

Rather than blame your body for malfunctioning, take a step back and ask yourself if you have put your body in the best possible environment to heal itself? Imagine how it feels to actually be inside your physical body. What is your body telling you? If you know you have a bad back and you keep lifting box after box, is your body going to feel burdened? Is your Celiac's disease going to be excited you ate gluten? Does your body feel loved and nurtured?

Be kind to yourself, even if you think you are doing everything you can think of. Your body is telling you that something needs a little more attention. This is an incredible gift. Rather than throw that gift on the garbage heap, take the time and have the openness to learn what that gift may be telling you.

FORGIVE YOUR SELF-CRITIC

Every day is filled with decisions, decisions and more decisions. You do the best you can with the info you have available and then – bam! The voice chimes that asks, "Why did you make that choice? What on earth possessed you to choose that? What the hell were you thinking?" Ah, the Peanut Gallery – aka, Mr. Inner Critic – has made an appearance.

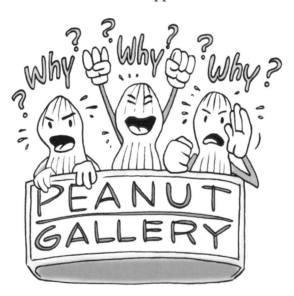

My advice: never take a second-guessing from a joker without fighting back. Stand up for yourself and all those choices made. You did the best you could with the info you had available. All those choices have led you to this moment right now. Instead of pining for a do-over, get out of your swirl of thoughts and root yourself here. Now. Be present and allow for some spontaneous awesomeness to happen.

All it takes is one conscious moment for an entire internal revolution to happen. And being berated by the self-critic does not count as being fully present. The self-critic is either obsessed with stuff that happened earlier or its fears about what may happen in the future. You wouldn't want to miss your enlightenment moment(s) because your energy was diverted by the self-critic.

FORGIVE YOUR PARENTS

Sometimes parents, caretakers, or guardians are awful. But, at some point, we have to forgive. I assume that everyone is doing the best they can given a parent or guardian's disposition, education, values, etc. These people have done the best that they were capable of at any given time. While you may have the desire to shame and berate and yell at them for not knowing any better, none of those things will get you very far. All you can control now is yourself and how you remember and respond to toxic energy in your body.

The time has come to stop being so reactive to how we think we should have been raised. The time has come to be grateful for being alive, to have another moment on this gorgeous planet to choose how we interact with the next moment. Forgiving our parents and dropping our stories about the past frees us up to decide more consciously about how we want to live. Old woe-is-me habits can die hard, so if unpleasant memories or angry thoughts arise, decide how you want to respond.

If you need to vent, find a safe place to do so. If you want to be ensnared in stories about the past, commit to that 100%. Be conscious that you are allowing your future decisions to be based entirely on unsettled accounts from your past. Which would you rather: continue to live in a state of reactivity and fear or unlearn and rewrite your history and live in love?

FORGIVE YOUR DOCTORS

Like parents, some doctors are awful. With authority figures, we like to assume that they are omniscient and have our best interests at heart, but that doesn't necessarily translate into the perfect care and treatment. Maybe your doctor was just having a bad day. Or maybe they are entirely incompetent. Either way, your doctor is going on with his/her life. Why are you filling up with toxic energy thinking about how you would like to punish/revenge/tell them off? How does harboring that resentment help you heal? Forgive your doctors. Bad diagnosis, misdiagnosis, poor treatment, and terrible bedside manner are just some of the reasons people tend to get so emotional about their healthcare providers.

Forgive your doctor and reclaim the present moment. Take back your power and possibility for great health by removing the energy from your memory of your diagnosis/bad treatment day.

FORGIVE YOUR ENVIRONMENT

When you moved to the area you live, you might have decided to locate there because it was convenient or affordable, or both. Over time, you may have found out that the water was poisoned, the air is toxic, or there is mold. I said it before: you made the best decision you could with the information that you had available. But, all of those choices about where and how we live add up. They add to make up who we are. We can't control what happened in our environment in the past, but we can certainly work towards making it different for the future.

Thinking that we are separate from our environment is a modern-day joke. Air conditioning, stronger buildings, and food at the grocery store all give the illusion that we have control and are independent from environmental variables. However, this is not the case. With the onslaught of laboratory generated chemicals such as food additives, fluoride, vaccines, and genetically modified everything, along with a lack of labeling so we know exactly what is in our food and where it comes from, this 'controlling the environment' hubris is saturating our body with unnatural chemicals. While we may not freeze to death, we are arguably now more susceptible to manmade environmental damages than ever before.

Become your own best friend, protector, and advocate. While we want to believe the government has our best interest at heart, we don't want to assume anything. Become an activist on your own behalf. Start transforming any energy you're wasting hating on stuff and channeling it to creating the reform you want.

FORGIVE GOD

This is very closely aligned with the entitlement to a healthy body. If we feel entitled to such a life, many believe it is God who grants it. So, if you believe in a God or gods or Holy Spirit, make sure you forgive them also if you feel you've been wronged. My basic premise is that you wanted life and chose to be here. Don't resent the entities that helped make that happen.

And drop the entitlements. Rather than praying for this or that and that and this and on and on, simply change your prayer to one of gratitude. "Thank you for this life." "Thank you for my great health and for being alive." Gratitude is much better for your energy than wanting like a spoiled little kid.

GIVE

Give love, forgiveness, gratitude, joy, a smile, a helping hand, an ear to listen, or a space to just feel safe and be. Give back to charity, find shelters or organizations that work with groups who are less fortunate. Sometimes the best way to get out of our incessant stories is to roll up our sleeves and get involved in activities happening in the moment. There is nothing like giving back to help realize how fortunate and how grateful we can be for the life we have.

ADD SOME SPICE

READ: *Count Your Blessings: 63 Things to Be Grateful for in Everyday Life . . . and How to Appreciate Them* by Robert Bly. When you actively acknowledge them, you'll realize you have more blessings in your life than problems. Other books to consider: *WORDS OF GRATITUDE: For Mind, Body and Soul; LIVING LIFE AS A THANK YOU: The Transformative Power of Daily Gratitude* and Louise L. Hay's *GRATITUDE: A Way of Life*

WATCH: The award-winning documentary Happy, about our most valued emotion. *http://www.thehappymovie.com/*

COMPARE: your list of stuff you're grateful for to this list of 60 things: *http://tinybuddha.com/blog/60-things-to-be-grateful-for-in-life/*

DO: start a Gratitude Journal. Whatever makes you happy…and grateful. And spend some time each day adding to it. *Gratitude: A Journal* by Catherine Price is a diary that contains exercises for you to try at the bottom of every other page and is filled with good quotes as you think about and record three positive moments from your day. Plus the small size is perfect for tossing in your bag or the drawer of your desk.

DOWNLOAD: *WHAT IS GRATITUDE? How to Attain an Attitude of Gratitude* BY D.L. Hart. A child's laughter, your cat's contented purring or perhaps your dog happily wagging their tail. What about the fact it's beautiful and sunny out, or the crickets are out in force, singing. Then there are beautiful flowers to appreciate, maybe the fact you got a good night's sleep or that lovely hug a friend just shared. Maybe it's a great movie, beautiful music… So many things to be grateful for, so little time.

CHILAX: while you give thanks with *Gratitude: Relaxing Native American Flute Music* 60 minutes of flowing waves and a slightly mystical (in the good way) feel.

ENTRAIN: your brain. Or at least accost it in the nicest way possible with subliminal messages of gratitude. *Gratitude Subliminal one* by "Dr. Virtual" on YouTube is around 25 minutes of pleasant bird sounds and nature'y noises, underneath which (use headphones for best results) you hear a gazillion messages of why you're thankful and grateful.

VOLUNTEER: One of the easiest ways to realize how good we have it is by working with others less fortunate. Try volunteering. Teach someone a special skill, work in a soup kitchen or other outreach facility, or just give your time and attention a la Big Brothers and Big Sisters.

SUMMARY

Be Grateful

- Saying 'Thank-You' is one of the most powerful phrases you can say.
- Gratitude lessens negativity and increases receptivity.

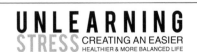

- Search out your held resentments and rather than hate them, practice being grateful.
- Forgiveness opens the door to more gratitude. Gratitude allows for more internal emotional and physical freedom.

FOOD FOR THOUGHT FOR CHAPTER 5

Make a list of all the events or people that you feel have somehow done you wrong in your life. Go thru that list and cultivate a feeling of gratitude for each of them. Whisper to yourself a 'thank you' to each of them. Without their actions or the sequence of events, you wouldn't be here right now, on the cusp of another moment, another breath, on this planet.

Go back to the list you made following Chapter 2 and look at all those things that triggered your fight or flight reaction. Say thank-you to all of those as well. Even if you can't feel gratitude at first, go thru the process of saying thank you. Fake the feeling at first if you must.

Gratitude can be hard to come by when we feel entitled to having life turn out a certain way. Make a list of your entitlements. What are all the things you feel you deserve? Those things that when the universe doesn't provide them can trigger you with grief, anger, doubt, frustration, anxiety, etc.

How does being beholden to these expectations, these entitlements, make your life any better? Or is this getting in your way? Do the things on this list take away your ability to be present and peaceful? Learn to be grateful for life as it is and own your power to make the next moment a little bit better or different from the previous if you need.

Chapter # 6 : Be Connected

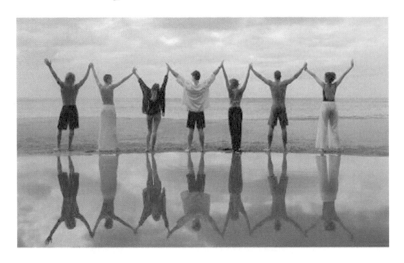

"Taoism is one of the world's only major religions in which food and sex are considered important paths to enlightenment."

— Kenneth Cohen, Qigong Master and author of *The Way of Qigong:* The Art and Science of Chinese Energy Healing

Good, nurturing, quality connections with people are so lacking right now that we collectively spend in excess of $82 billion annually for anti-anxiety meds, anti-depressants, stimulants and pricey anti-psychotic drugs. "What you find with them when you look at long term outcomes," notes science journalist and author Robert Whitaker, "you see more people having chronic symptoms long term than you do in the unmedicated."[66]

Not all of this dependence on drugs will be remedied by a quality chat, but, better connections with living things—be they human, four-legged and fuzzy, or arboreal and flowering, undoubtedly changes our energy.

A recent 30+ year study that followed more than 800 children into adulthood tracked a variety of factors such as how much a child was liked, how much time they spent with peers in activities like youth groups and sports clubs and whether they had a solid foundation of social connectedness. The youngsters with positive social relationships grew to be adults who were better adjusted and happier, regardless of socioeconomic factors. In cases where this pathway

UNLEARNING STRESS CREATING AN EASIER HEALTHIER & MORE BALANCED LIFE

of youth interpersonal connection was weak, adult wellbeing turned out similarly lacking.[67]

Feeling socially isolated also turns out to compromise another key ingredient in your health: a good night's sleep. "Loneliness has been associated with adverse effects on health," explains one researcher at the University of Chicago who discovered that people who felt lonely woke up more during the night.

> *Feeling socially isolated also turns out to compromise another key ingredient in your health: a good night's sleep.*

"The relationship between loneliness and restless sleep appears to operate across the range of perceived connectedness."[68] Feelings of loneliness have been linked to poor health,[69] higher levels of stress,[70] sub-par brain function[71] and are possibly even contagious.[72]

People who feel lonely are also:

…   prone to obesity (in part because they're less likely to exercise).

…   more likely to die after a serious operation.

…   plagued with more hormonal imbalances, internal inflammation and memory decline.

…   given to depression and inferior cognitive function.[73]

Feeling lonely alters how we function at the most fundamental level, including gene expression (epigenetics). "When you are lonely," writes Stephen Marche in an in-depth piece on the topic in *The Atlantic*, "your whole body is lonely."[74] And yet, more of us are disconnected, isolated, and lonely. When researchers ask people "How often do you feel you are 'in tune' with the people around you?" and "How often do you feel you lack companionship?" The answers reveal a rising tide of loneliness.

In the US, for example, in 1950, a scant 1 in 10 households were made up of the loneliest number: 1. 60 years later that number has almost tripled.[75] Between 1985 and 2004, the number of people reporting that they had no one to discuss anything of importance with rose from 10% to 25%. The rise in loneliness seems to be continuing unabated to the point where health care professionals across the world have begun to refer to it as an epidemic.

Why would this be in this age of 24/7 Social Media connectedness?

Digital only social connections mean we also miss out on the physical contact of rubbing shoulders, shaking hands, smelling perfumes, and mirroring expressions that happen with in-person gatherings. Digital contact eliminates the most tactile and sensuously delicious experiences, reducing them to the basest of visual cues and cognitive merry go-rounds.

The initial lesson that my first Native American teacher ever taught me was that humans are no better than every other thing on the planet. By 'thing' that meant everything: insects, birds, fish, rocks, trees, weeds, shrubs, clouds, rain, dirt, etc. The teacher continued to say that not only are we no better than, we are also entirely connected to all those things. We are all part of the same giant web of interconnectedness, whether we like it or not.

When Buddha is depicted in sunny mood, it's because he understood the secret power of smiling and laughing.

The effect of this teaching moves us from being on top of a food and social hierarchy, to being more horizontal, where we are respectful of all life. This idea of already being connected also makes it easier to receive spiritual and emotional nourishment from your environment. If you believe the trees and rocks can enhance your energy, then every walk you take or every time you consciously focus on the nature, your energetic response is magnified. But if you see nature as something to be conquered or inconsequential, then you are confined to finding connections only with other conquerors: humans.

CONNECT WITH A PET

When asked who they talk to when they get upset, for many children, it's their pet. "This points to the importance of pets as a source of comfort and developing empathy," explains child-development expert Dr. James Griffin. Pets are not only man's best friend, they can also help you make more friends of the two-legged persuasion. Walking the dog tends to lead to more conversations and in turn, more social connectedness, which means living a longer, healthier life with less mental or physical decline.

UNLEARNING STRESS CREATING AN EASIER HEALTHIER & MORE BALANCED LIFE

"Compared to walking alone," adds Dr. Sandra Barker, director of the Center for Human-Animal Interaction at Virginia Commonwealth University, "it's hard to walk a dog and not have someone talk or interact with you...I think we're just at the tip of the iceberg in terms of what we know about the human-animal bond and its potential health benefits," she continues. "This area is primed for a lot of research that still needs to be done."

Just think, while Fido's getting his/her walk, you'll be improving your heart health. Dog people have much better post-heart attack survival rates, recovering faster when the things go haywire, lowering your heart and blood pressure. And by being more physically active, you're less likely to become obese, and all that walking will pay off in terms of staying mobile as you age.[76]

Don't own a dog? Don't let that stop you. You can always rent one from a service like FlexPets in California and NYC or Tokyo's Janet Village.[77] Or, better yet, why not volunteer at your local animal shelter to walk some of their dogs? "If you are feeling a little lonely," adds Gary Patronek, of the Animal Rescue League of Boston, "we are here."[78]

CONNECT WITH LAUGHTER

Charlie Chaplin once observed: "A day without laughter is a day wasted." Laugher really is the best medicine in so many ways, starting with how it quiets the fight/flight response and lowers your levels of stress hormones. Think about it: should you happen to find yourself being chased by a tiger, about the last thing you'll be doing is have a good belly laugh. When you laugh, you get to enjoy those feel-good endorphins which your body releases after a rewarding activity. Now you are the one chasing the tiger away!

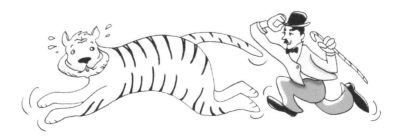

Western medicine is doing more research looking at why laughter has such beneficial physiologic effects. It is a universal physiologic and psychological response that almost all people – and some animals – can relate to, which is why it has been shown to have a huge impact on mental stress and possibly even help ameliorate the risk of heart disease.[79]

So if you're feeling a bit rough around the edges, connect through the power of laughter. Try Netflixing or Hulu'ing a funny movie. Read an author who cracks you up. Or just simply laugh. "Laughter Yoga" and "laughter meditation" are gaining popularity throughout the world. "Imagine a humorous situation, remember funny jokes, or think about how odd it is to be laughing by yourself," advises DailyOM. "When the giggles start to rise, let them. Let the laughter ripple through your belly and down into the soles of your feet. Let the laughter lead to physical movement. Roll on the floor, if you have to, and keep on laughing until you stop."[80]

CONNECT WITH SOMEONE ELSE

Sex makes life more fun.

And it can also improve your health.

One of the most important things that happen in the body when we couple up is the hormone oxytocin gets activated. Oxytocin responds to physical touch, helping babies and mothers bond during breastfeeding. Oxytocin is also very active during intercourse. Oxytocin increases with nipple and genital stimulation, but it can also increase just by thinking about someone you love. When oxytocin levels are high, we feel less anxiety, more trust, and less stress.

The Taoists didn't necessarily know anything about oxytocin, but that didn't stop them from figuring out how to maximize enjoyment and health through sex.

The Taoists didn't necessarily know anything about oxytocin, but that didn't stop them from figuring out how to maximize enjoyment and health through sex. They have taken their appreciation for sex and have interwoven it with their approach to life, wellness, and aging. In the Chinese medicine worldview, there is a concept called Jing, or "essence".

This Jing was so important in our life process, they considered it to be the "primordial seed" that begets most other energies of life. When Jing is strong, so is your health, stamina, ability to age well and overall quality of life. But, being deficient in Jing is said to cause everything from infertility, aging less gracefully and generally feeling lousy.

The quality of our Jing comes a lot from our parents. So if you were blessed with strong and healthy parents and had a relatively uncomplicated delivery, you were probably blessed with good amounts of Jing. But if you were premature, had weak parents, or grew up in a toxic environment, your Jing may have been compromised.

The good news: we can ration our Jing, and potentially even enhance it, thru good lifestyle habits and practicing the Taoist art of sex and lovemaking.

The gist of this Taoist sexual practice is fully committing to the present moment and being as aware of as many senses as possible. Take time to luxuriate in the touch of your partner. Foreplay, caressing, massage, kissing, all help to activate the Qi. After the foreplay, the focus on the Tao of sex diverges depending on your gender.

Brace yourself.

Are you ready?

If you're female, Taoist sexual practices encourage as many orgasms as possible.

But if you're male, there's a twist: men are encouraged to orgasm often, but they have to be more judicious about their frequency of ejaculation. As the teaching goes, the two, ejaculation and orgasm, can be separated.

MEN and JING: In the Taoist context, ejaculation = energy spent. This brings to mind a fun French phrase, La petite mort, a euphemism for male orgasm that translates as "the little death."

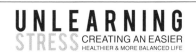

The classical Tao of Sex books are filled with great quotes and guidelines about how much is too much ejaculation. For our purposes, after a man ejaculates, he should feel energized, and not exhausted.

There is a huge distinction here between sex and ejaculation. This practice recommends having sex as much as possible, which allows for even more connection. But men must temper their ejaculation. There is even an art of energy cultivation that teaches a man how to orgasm without ejaculation. This is part of the advanced course! In the beginning, avoid that point of no return, focus on moving the energy back up into the body, and stop before ejaculating. "Blue balls" usually won't happen, or if there is discomfort, it usually won't stay for long. Plus, you'll find that you are stronger, hornier, and more present in your day to day as your Jing is activated and flowing throughout your body, rather than losing it in a fleeting moment of ecstasy.

WOMEN and JING: For women, the Taoist idea of having as many orgasms as possible is a way of staying connected with the sexual organs so the energy doesn't become blocked. Free flowing and strong energy lays the foundation for health and freedom. Blocked, unfulfilled, and stagnant energy is the precursor of disease. This notion of women surrendering to the moment as much as possible is showing up more often as women practice getting in touch with their power.

The woman-as-goddess author[81] and personality, Mama Gena leads Sister Goddess workshops. Here she helps women get comfortable with their lady parts, as in get out a hand mirror and take a good long look below. By teaching the ladies to tap into their inner "pussy power", she helps them to feel sexy, empowered and learn how to "conjure" their desires.

Seriously. An important part of the Sister Goddess curriculum involves a lot of self-pleasuring and then bragging about the happy fallout to the other Sister Goddess in class the next week. The more orgasms a woman has, says the apparent Tao-of-Sexy Mama G, the more she can conjure everything her heart desires: from gorgeous clothes to jewelry to great contacts that lead to new jobs and career growth.

For both sexes, though, the main takeaway is this: making love consciously and wisely is a vital way to connect. It makes stagnant energy fields flow again, and the free exchange of energy can both heal and even lead to mutual enlightenment. Or, at the very least, be a tasty afternoon delight.

ADD SOME SPICE

READ: *Mama Gena's School of Womanly Arts: Using the Power of Pleasure to Have Your Way with the World; The Tao of Love and Sex* by Jolan Chang, *The Tao of Love, Sex, and Longevity* by Daniel P. Reid

LAUGH: http://www.laughteryoga.org/

LISTEN: Groovify your general environment with good music. Pandora is like having your own DJ who understands what you like and has exquisite taste and creates a custom soundtrack to your life.

FOR FUN: *Naked* and *Me Talk Pretty Some Day* by David Sedaris; *Calvin and Hobbes* by Bill Watterson

WATCH: something hilarious! A super-fun project would be to stream or rent your way through Time Out London's list of the *Top 100 Best Comedy Movies* as chosen by a pack of comedy writers, actors, directors and fan. While some are an acquired taste, some or more culty, many are just excellent, including *Young Frankenstein, Borat, Annie Hall, Groundhog Day, Shaun of the Dead, The Big Lebowski, The Blues Brothers, Blazing Saddles* and *This is Spinal Tap.*

MEDITATE: on connecting. Assume your ideal meditation position and do your deep breathing. Once your shoulders are relaxed and your body is feeling good, imagine yourself at the center of a giant web. In the first ring of the web, see your friends and family. See also the trees outside your home or office. Put your pets, neighborhood birds, or other wildlife in that first ring also. Then, expand the web to the second ring to include your more distant relatives and your friend's friends. Expand the web to then include everyone in your state or country. Keep going with your web until you are connected with every living thing in the world. Imagine how you might act and behave if you could be conscious of this connection all the time.

DO: Why not send someone wonderful a gift just because? What a wonderful way to connect. Plus if it makes them chuckle or laugh, you get extra brownie points. Two great places to score offbeat gifts include Archie McPhee (www.mcphee.com)- Bacon bandages, rubber chicken-head masks and plastic Bavarian lederhosen that hop about and yodel (the remote control looks like a knockwurst); and ThinkGeek (www.thinkgeek.com) with Star Wars Family decals for the back window of the car; Doctor Who Tardis cookie jar that talks; and zombie soap.

SUMMARY

Chapter 6: Be Connected

- Loneliness can be damaging to your health.

- Realize your connection with all things by removing the thinking that we are better than anything else.

- Increase your connections by getting a pet, volunteering, or simply having more aware sex.

FOOD FOR THOUGHT FOR CHAPTER 6

Think about all that has happened over the course of your life that has helped to make this moment possible for you.

When was the last time you laughed out loud—a lot?

What are your strongest social connections? Do they support you? How do you feel supported? Do they know you appreciate them?

What are your weakest connections that you wish were stronger? Are there steps you can take to make them stronger? What are those steps?

Make a list of all the things or people you feel you are better than. How does this list make you feel? How much energy did you put in to constantly feel better than them? Does this list or feelings help you feel more connected or less? Does feeling superior improve or hinder your ability to be in the moment?

Chapter # 7 : Be Active

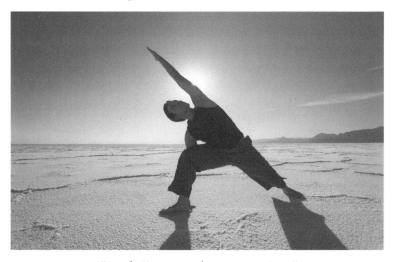

"Lord, I've got to keep on moving."

— Bob Marley

There is an ongoing debate among archaeologists about how ancient people moved around and populated the world. We can likely figure that a combination of geographical and sociological pressures had a lot to say about how and why people moved the way they did. But if we look at our modern tendencies, it strikes me as being entirely reasonable that some people just had an itch for adventure.

The population of Polynesia is one of the most interesting questions. Some of the latest genetic research suggests that Polynesians can be traced back to Asia and Taiwan. The exact route taken and length of time for these people to spread across the Pacific to Polynesia is not 100% agreed upon, but whether they moved quickly like an "Express Train", more leisurely "Slow Boat" style, or meandering, "Entangled Bank" model, the fact is, these people moved.[82]

Great distances.

Whether studying the tides, building boats, hunting, fishing, or dancing, moving and understanding movement is critical to the Polynesian way of life. And it needs to be critical to yours in order to fully actualize your potential in the human form. Movement is the basis of living – literally, starting with eggs, sperm, cell division and expansion. A life without movement is no life at all.

According to Chinese Medicine, quality movement is so important it has its own special symbol: the Tai ji/yin yang symbol.

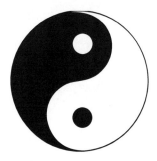

Where Yin is dark, solid, flat, inward, decreasing, and tranquil, Yang is light, heat, stimulation, arousal, movement. You can think of Yin as the shade to Yang's sunny side of the street. Yang is potential and Yin its completion. As Yin turns back into Yang and Yang into Yin, the result is an ongoing ebb and flow of creation and destruction; renewal and decay.

This tension is what holds the entire universe in place. Because the symbol is based on the idea of non-stop movement, the lines between the two halves aren't straight: they're curved. In other words, this symbol is visual shorthand for the dynamic movement – and resulting tension – that holds everything in the universe in place, from the planets all the way down to our microscopic cells.

Think of each cell as containing both the seeds of perfect health and its polar opposite: disease. So if the balance of yin and yang within becomes distorted, or the movement between them is blocked, we start to feel slow, sluggish, or lousy. However, the good news is that no matter how diseased a particular cell or organ or tissue of your body might be, the seeds of manifesting health are always energetically present according to this yin/yang theory.

Health and balance has to constantly be achieved, one moment to the next. There is no static finish line of 'health'. How well we are able to achieve this balance moment after moment depends on the internal mental and physical milieu we create.

In Chinese medicine thought, your feelings of stress, and their subsequent symptoms, are simply a manifestation of an imbalance of the yin and yang in the body. Change the imbalance and you change your experience of the stress. And changing this disharmony demands movement.

When Yin and Yang shift back and forth, they generate another form of energy. This friction is similar to what happens when you rub your hands together to create heat. In this Chinese medicine worldview, the byproduct of the perpetual volleying between Yin and Yang is the "gas" that fuels the engines of our existence, the energy that sustains each and every one of us, that keeps our blood flowing where it's supposed to, called Qi (pronounced "chee"). [83]

While we all tend to talk about a single "Qi", in truth, there are a number of aspects to Qi. Looking at blood, for instance, Qi is said to generate it, move it and hold it in the vessels. These functions allude to the larger actions of Qi which include functions like: transform, transport, hold, raise, protect and keep you warm – like a protective cocoon. And like a protective cocoon, when the conditions are right, Qi performs all these tasks to create a beautiful and healthy you.

To create ideal conditions for your Qi to flourish, we have to put ourselves in an environment where we feel nurtured. Everything that makes us who we are is connected to everything else. The beauty of everything being connected is you can change input anywhere into the mind/body/spirit cycle and the entire mechanism is affected. This connectivity is also the bummer because it means 'compartmentalization' is an illusion. And for this chapter, this means that you can't sit on the couch all day and expect to have unlimited energy.

> *"In the Tao, it is written*
>
> *First there was the eternal Tao*
>
> *From the Tao came One*
>
> *From One came Two*
>
> *From Two came Three*
>
> *From Three came ten thousand other things."*
>
> *- Tao Te Ching*

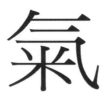

The Chinese character for Qi has a lower radical that stands for "grain" and an upper radical for "rising vapor"; together, these radicals give the idea of cooking grain and distilling its essence. Distilling the essence of your Qi, keeping it happy if you will, relies on the proper internal and external conditions: movement.

If the Qi is prevented from moving, if it gets sluggish, stagnant or blocked, we feel terrible. Stuck Qi is unhappy Qi and tends to manifest with imbalances ranging from full-on disease to the less dire, but equally frustrating, feelings of fatigue, exhaustion and being stuck and unmotivated. And usually when you feel this way, the last thing you want to do is get moving. But this is in fact exactly what you need to be doing.

Even with conditions like cancer, the traditional medical advice to rest after treatment has finally been proved wrong. "Traditionally doctors and nurses have often advised patients to rest during chemotherapy and radiotherapy or after cancer treatment," explains Professor Robert Thomas, a consulting oncologist at Addenbrookes and Bedford Hospitals in the UK. "In this case, however, rest is not best. A common side effect of cancer treatment, such as chemotherapy, is fatigue, which leads to reduction in mood, maybe anxiety and ultimately depression."

Not only does regular exercise during cancer treatments significantly improve mood and psychological wellbeing, it can help stave off the frustrating concentration and memory problems that can occur after treatment, dubbed "chemo brain."[84]

"Physical activity helps patients in a number of really good ways," continues Thomas. "It reduces the side effects of treatment, it makes patients feel better and more recently, it has been shown that regular exercise after cancer will actually reduce your risk of relapse and improve your overall chance of living a healthy, long life."[85]

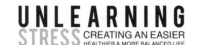

Similarly, a recent study shows that heart patients may also benefit from exercise that is vigorous, that is to say 85-95% of your maximum. When patients at cardiac rehab centers in Norway who worked out vigorously were compared with the patients who exercised at moderate intensity, 60-70% of maximum, there was virtually no difference between the rates of post-workout heart malfunctions. In fact, the results were strong enough that the lead researcher of the study, published in the medical journal Circulation[86], felt compelled to add: "I think (high intensity training) should be considered for patients with coronary heart disease."[87]

Exercise…

- … improves your body's ability to clean cellular house of damaged or degraded tissue;[88]
- … is thought to reduce the risk of breast cancer (even mild physical activity);[89]
- … can dramatically reduce the risk of Type 2 diabetes;[90]
- … has been shown to improve the health of people living with chronic kidney disease;[91]
- … gives frail seniors a new lease on life (both physically and cognitively) after just three months;[92]
- … alleviates pain, especially from nerve damage by reducing small signaling molecules called cytokines that promote inflammation;[93]
- … reduces anxiety, improving your response to emotional events;[94]
- … enables you to get a better night's sleep;[95]
- … and fights depression, improves your mood and can even improve self-esteem, social skills and your ability to think.[96]

Physiologically, movement promotes health in two key ways, by:

1. **Reducing oxidative damage** – a byproduct of combining the food we burn for energy with the oxygen we breathe, which, in excess, leaves a trail of damage not unlike rust on a metal such as iron;[97]

2. **Dampening inflammation.**

 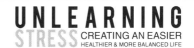

Together, oxidative damage and inflammation are the Dastardly Duo of the health world, responsible for many modern diseases of deterioration, including Alzheimer's and Parkinson's, heart disease and atherosclerosis, cancer, inflammatory bowel disease, osteoarthritis and osteoporosis and rheumatoid arthritis.

So you have two choices: (1) sit on your butt too much and congratulations: you've virtually doubled your risk of degenerative disease. Or (2) set aside time to exercise, which then entitles you a Good Housekeeping Karma award for honoring the temple that is your body.

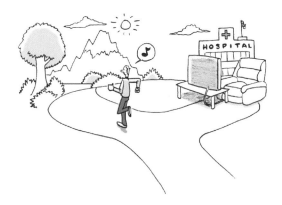

As a rule of thumb, the better your aerobic capacity, the better your health. "Low aerobic exercise capacity is a strong predictor of premature morbidity and mortality in both healthy adults and people with cardiovascular disease," explain researchers from the Norwegian University of Science and Technology's KG Jebsen Center of Exercise in Medicine who were testing the idea that the better shape your ticker is in, the longer you are likely to live the good life. "In the elderly, poor performance on treadmill- or extended walking tests indicates proximity to future health decline."[98]

These insights aren't exactly new. Chinese medicine has said to keep moving. And another famous guy from a couple thousand years ago noted something similar: "Lack of activity destroys the good condition of every human being," noted Plato almost 2,500 years ago, "while movement and methodical physical exercise save it and preserve it."

In other words: Use it…or lose it.

EXERCISE YOUR BRAWN

Our resident exercise expert, exercise physiologist Jeff Dolgan, says if you want to live your best life possible, there are four types of exercise you should do: cardio, weights, flexibility and maintaining your motor skills such as balance and coordination. According to the Mayo Clinic, as little as 30 minutes a day is all it takes and this can even be something as simple and enjoyable as walking briskly. Adding some weight-training two to three times weekly confers even more benefits, in particular helping to maintain bone health.[99]

These are the exercise guidelines provided by the American College of Sports Medicine: [100]

CARDIO: Plan to spend about 2.5 hours per week exercising at moderate intensity, be it concentrated in 2-3 bouts of vigorous activity each lasting 20-60 minutes, like aerobics, running, biking or interval training. Or you can spread it out over 5 days for a half hour of something moderate like brisk walking. Or, you can really spread it out into 10 minute sessions whenever you have a break in your schedule. The goal is to get your weekly total to 150 minutes.

WEIGHT TRAINING: Spend 2-3 days each week resistance-training your major muscle groups: your legs, stomach, arms, back and shoulders. The ACSM advises that you allow 48 hours to pass between sessions so your muscles can proper recover and become stronger.

> *Cardio, Weights, Flexibility, and Neuromotor training are the 4 major types of exercise. A well-rounded program includes exercises for each of them.*

FLEXIBILITY: Increase your flexibility by stretching your muscles 2-3 times a week to the point where they start to get tight and then hold that for around 30 seconds. Repeating each stretch 2-4 times until you end up hitting 60 seconds per stretch.

NEUROMOTOR: Make sure 2-3 of your workouts each week improve your functional fitness by doing activities like tai chi and yoga.

EXERCISE YOUR OPTIONS

Start small - with whatever areas of life you feel are stagnant. Do you always drive the same route? Wear your watch on the same wrist? Brush your teeth with the same hand? Then it's time to switch it up, taking a different route home or using your awkward wrist or hand. When you change your routine, you make something "new" again. In order to process the change, your brain has to activate new neurons.

Flowing Qi isn't going to happen without you doing your part, so rather than emailing, walk over to chat with that co-worker, take the dog for a walk on a different route, and instead of working all the time, take a vacation, even a staycation will do. Beautiful, flowing, dynamic Qi is what you want, but for that to happen, you need to move. And not just physically, but mentally as well. Once you get moving, you'll see how Qi begets more Qi. And when this happens, congrats, you've begun to rewrite the Story of You.

EXERCISE YOUR RESOLVE

When you practice Sitting (Chapter #3), really try to be active about identifying all pathological cravings, incessant thoughts and long-held resentments that collectively are blocking your Qi. By observing them, you can change them and unblock the flow across your mind/body/spirit, enabling the Qi to be created, balanced, harmonized and fully expressed.

EXERCISE YOUR ENZYMES

Ben Franklin and Thomas Jefferson changed the world standing up. Literally. Both used "standing" desks because sitting for extended periods does such bad things to your health. Starting with the size of your butt. Sitting suppresses the main molecule responsible for breaking down fat, an enzyme called lipase. When lipase is active, your body can burn fat for fuel, but sitting for long stretches flips the lipase switch to "off".[101] Also worse for wear is your heart; sitting for more than 6 hours a day increases your risk of heart disease a whopping 64%. Ditto your chances of getting cancer and your cholesterol levels.

In all, sitting too much steals a good seven or more years from your lifespan. Plus, even if you work out diligently a full hour every day, being seated the rest of the day is not sufficient for reversing the risks associated with so much sitting.[102] So if you're watching your kid's soccer game, do it standing up. Get in the habit of standing up every 15 minutes and at least once an hour. Make a habit of taking phone calls standing up, and maybe even invest in a treadmill desk.

EXERCISE YOUR NAVIGATION SKILLS

Whether from eating undercooked meat, being careless with the cat litter or all manner of other things life throws your way, almost all of us have had an infection at some point. These range from the virus that causes cold sores (HSV-1) and Cytomegalovirus (CMV) which at least 60% of the US population has, to toxoplasmosis, found in similar percentages internationally.

Even ear infections you had as a kid can take a residual toll on your balance as an adult as falls are one of the top causes of death in the elderly. However, there is something you can do about it: recalibrate the connection between your brain and your body.

"The brain maintains "maps" of the body," explains Paul Jaminet, co-author of *Perfect Health Diet: Four Steps to Renewed Health, Youthful Vitality and Long Life*. As your body changes, your mental map must incorporate the changes as well. If your body is capable of performing a task, it may not be able to if your brain and body are so out of synch. "As a result," continues Jaminet, "the brain may believe a movement is impossible or dangerous and block its performance."

To update your brain map, you need to move in a way that reassures your brain that what you're asking it to do isn't "dangerous". How? By training in a way that's slow and deliberate. Good options for this include yoga, Qi Gong and Tai Chi. Experiment to see what kind of movement you enjoy most and feel best balances your Qi.

 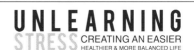

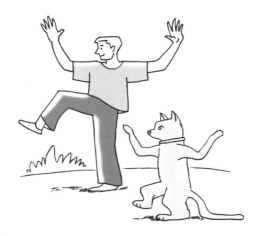

EXERCISE YOUR EMERGENCY EXIT POTENTIAL

If you had to run for your life, could you? Fight off a predator? Scale a barricade? Sprint up a hill? Cling to a branch in a flood? "Next time you are at the gym and you see all the men and women plodding away on the cross-trainer or pushing weights on a machine with poor technique, ask yourself whether you think they could get out of a similar situation," observes Jamie Scott, nutrition, sports- and exercise-medicine and fitness expert with an impressive array of expert letters to his name.[103] "Better yet, ask them if they think they could…I would argue that having power in your body gives one the power of belief in your mind."[104]

If you train mindlessly, it might be time to reevaluate why. The thought of "plodding away" for hours on a treadmill sounds anything but inspiring. The best exercise is the one you'll do for the rest of your life and that challenges you not just in body, but mind, too … and maybe even your evacuation superpowers. It even appears that the US Army is changing the way they train, doing away with the standard pushup and pull-up and getting more dynamic and functional.[105]

EXERCISE YOUR MAMA'S ADVICE

Stand up straight. Walking, sitting properly, and just moving around in proper alignment eliminates untold amounts of stress and daily wear and tear

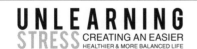

on your body. The Alexander Technique is a method of unlearning bad physical habits and relearning how to hold your head correctly and distribute your weight evenly. This technique has been shown to alleviate any number of uncomfortable conditions, including minor digestive issues, tension headaches and pain.

British researchers found that the Alexander technique offered significant long-term relief from chronic back pain.[106] As can a regular yoga practice.[107] Or the McKenzie Method if your back already hurts. And once you start to live in your body in alignment with the way it was designed, don't be surprised if you how you feel about yourself starts changing.

According to the Feldenkrais Method, a system of healing pain and overcoming limitations by moving correctly, any time you change how you move, you change your internal image of yourself. This, in turn, changes how you perceive yourself consciously. In other words: moving better = better self-image = change in conscious perception. "What I am after," noted Moshé Feldenkrais once about the goal of his eponymous system, "is more flexible minds, not just more flexible bodies."[108]

EXERCISE YOUR MOBILIZATION

To be truly mobile, your body needs to get all your various parts working in concert, from your muscles to your soft tissue, joints, motor control, range of motion and neuromotor skills. Trainer Kelly Starrett, DPT, has shot a massive library worth of helpful video-blogs at Mobility WOD (www.mobilitywod.com) that address everything from how to warm up for exercise properly to post-workout issues and what to do about them. Another great resource is my trainer, former Marine Special-Ops, Carlos Arias. Carlos has an online training program for at-home fitness program. You can find it here: http://www.animuscrossfit.com/foundations/

ADD SOME SPICE

SHIMMY: If you haven't yet incorporated regular movement into your life, you could start by getting your hula on with New Zealand-born fitness expert Anna-Rita Sloss. "Hot Hula is a blend of all the different Polynesian cultures coming together to the beat of drums to create a complete one-hour fitness workout," Sloss explains.[109] It promises to improve your abs and lower body, along with your sense of sensual fun. Available as a 3-DVD set from Anna-Rita.com.

HOP: out of the workout box. So you're feeling oh so been-there-done-that about your workouts. Here are some "offbeat" (um, okay, kinda weird) ones that might reignite your workout mojo.[110] If you live where it snows and can wait for winter, you can always harness up your pooch and let him/her pull you on your skis for a fun day of skijoring. Or combine your loves of spinning and singing as you pedal and sweat in a karaoke spin class. If singing the praises of the Almighty is more your speed, try Body Gospel, a "faith-based" workout with each workout beginning with a prayer set to gospel tunes. And summer fun in the sun wouldn't be complete without water and a beach ball, even better if it's big enough for you to fit inside it. Waterwalkerz are giant, transparent blow-up beach balls which float on the water's surface with you inside, engaging your abs, sense of balance and whatever else is necessary to stay upright and in motion.

READ: *SITTING KILLS, MOVING HEALS: How Everyday Movement Will Prevent Pain, Illness and Early Death – and Exercise Alone Won't* written by NASA scientist Joan Vernikos who was given the task of finding out why astronauts in the prime of life returned from space with weaker muscles, worse eyesight, poorer hearing and even lower levels of testosterone. One word: gravity. Spending time without it actually mirrors what happens to us as we age if we don't remain active. But according to Vernikos, it's surprisingly easy to fight back. In fact, the most beneficial activity you can do for your health is stand up every 15 minutes or so, and move around a lot throughout the day.

The Web That Has No Weaver by Ted Kaptchuk is a great book to understand the basics of Chinese medicine. You can read more about the different types of Qi and how they circulate thru the body.

ARISE: To remember to get up often from your computer, you can install a program to give you a needed nudge. If you're on Windows, try Workrave (www.workrave.org) while Mac users can download Time Out (http://www.dejal.com/timeout/). When it's time to stand

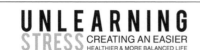

up, these programs dim your desktop to help pry your butt from your chair.[111]

WALK: while you're on the clock. A treadmill desk is one of the easiest ways to incorporate gentle movement into your work day. The TrekDesk (www.trekdesk.com) will accommodate most any treadmill, offers a lot of desk surface-space and folds up easily when you need to move it or store it. Enthusiastic users report losing up to a pound a week, and yes, it's safe to be on the move all day. Your cave-ancestors certainly were, logging about 30-35 miles per day.

COUNT: your steps. If you want to stay healthy, in addition to your workout or formal exercise, you need to get in at least 10,000 steps a day. Strapping on a pedometer is the easiest way to keep track. Some recommended ones include the Omron HJ-112, Yamax Digiwalker CW-701 and the much-loved Fitbit.[112]

BALANCE: Qi Gong or Tai Chi classes. There are several different kinds, so experiment with a variety to find the class that suits you the best. Often times local martial arts or yoga studios are a good place to look for these. If all else fails, I like the DVD *Qi Gong for Beginners* by Lee Holden and *Sunrise Tai Chi* by Ramel Rones.

SUMMARY

Be Active

- A critical component of all good health according to Chinese medicine is movement.
- Western medicine continues to show the benefits of adequate exercise in boosting metabolism, increasing energy, and decreasing the stress response.
- A balanced exercise regimen includes four types of movement: cardio, weights, flexibility and maintaining your motor skills (balance & coordination).

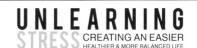

FOOD FOR THOUGHT FOR CHAPTER 7

Where are you the most stagnant in your life? Is it physically? Mentally? Emotionally? Spiritually?

If you had to make one change in your life that would make a difference in moving this stuck energy, what would it be?

Are there times where you chose to remain stuck/seated instead of moving that you came to regret?

If you need to work out more but you don't have the time, is there a way to create more time or to rethink your workout to make it easier to achieve your goals? Can you get up earlier? Can you do pushups during the day? Squats at home? Perhaps hire a trainer to give you a total program to fit your lifestyle?

Chapter # 8 : Be Visionary

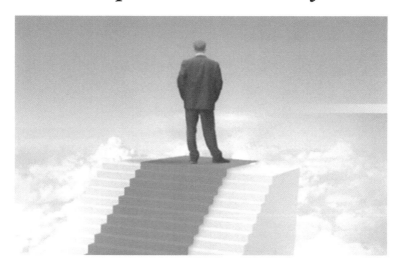

"Destiny is not a matter of chance, it is a matter of choice.
It is not a thing to be waited for, it is a thing to be achieved."

—William Jennings Bryan[113]

In the 1400's a big block of stone became the focus of a lot of attention. This hunk of marble was imported from Carrera and transported to Florence's cathedral of Santa Maria Del Fiore. Once there, it was to become a series of Old Testament sculptures adorning the buttresses. While many artists attempted to make headway with the marble behemoth, it continued to prove so troublesome that countless fits and starts later it was finally simply abandoned in the workshop yard. There it languished, unprotected and exposed to the elements for almost a century. In other words, an embarrassment of epic proportions.

Determined to finally turn the piece into something respectable, the Overseers of the Office of Works of the Duomo had it placed on its end and experts, including Leonardo da Vinci, were brought in.

However, it was a young 26-year old who won the commission.[114]

So why was Michelangelo able to beat out someone of da Vinci's stature to win this prestigious prize at such a tender age? How did he turn a colossal white elephant nicknamed The Giant, so daunting that it had successfully stymied fellow artists for almost 100 years, into the elegant, 17 foot tall masterpiece that is the David within just two years?

Probably because he was a man with a plan.

> *"In every block of marble I see a statue as plain as though it stood before me, shaped and perfect in attitude and action,"* Michelangelo once said. *"I have only to hew away the rough walls that imprison the lovely apparition to reveal it to the other eyes as mine see it."*

With the David as his destination, Michelangelo knew exactly what was waiting for expression within The Giant: i.e. where his journey was headed. As to how he got there: that wasn't set in stone (so to speak) but an organic process of chipping away whatever "doesn't look like David." And how did he know which parts of The Giant were not-David and which were? He had a crystal-clear vision of where he wanted to end up.

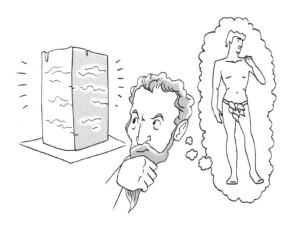

Whether you label it a vision or a goal or creativity, they're one and the same – knowing where you want to go. That is the "big secret" to success. Without vision, an idea for a killer script, the blueprints for a can't-lose product, or the potential for vibrant health, all remain just blocks of marble until the David-destination within is envisioned clearly. However, the more David-like your vision of what you want, the more glaring the contrast between where you are now and where you want to be. So what is your vision? Chances are in trying to answer this question, even more questions arise:

Does this job reflect how I want to be living?

Is this relationship nurturing to my healthy expression?

Am I spending my time each day meaningfully?

These are some pretty heavy questions. It takes courage to answer them honestly. And if your answer is "no" to any of them, this book is here to help. Are you killing yourself slowly by working harder and longer, fueling your body with junk instead of nourishing food, laughing less, stressing more and feeling angry with yourself and pretty much everyone else on the planet?

The choice to destroy ourselves at varying rates of speed can manifest in a variety of ways. Mental and emotional turmoil has the same detrimental energetic impact as substance abuse. Whether your vice is alcohol, heroine, caffeine, constant email checking, or panic attacks, it is time to take long hard look at that behavior and see if it fits into the larger vision you have for your life. Is self-combustion what you envisioned when thinking about making your David sculpture out of your life?

Not sure how to re-imagine your life? Let's start at the beginning. We believe that a desire to self-combust is completely at odds with our belief about the nature of life. Your spirit decided to be born. You wanted to be here. Your larger spirit decided it wanted to have a human to experience of life on Earth. This Earth isn't some kind of purgatory for the soul, but rather a play land of potential adventures and experiences. A spiritual amusement park if you will.

Don't ever doubt you wanted to be here because if you didn't, you wouldn't. Why struggle with life believing that this is a hard place to be? Or that your life here is to pay a penance for something that happened long ago? Delete that story from your psyche and replace it with the one that says this planet is possibly the most amazing place to be in the universe. So let's go and savor life to the fullest.

If you're stuck thinking life should be a struggle or that you are not worthy of being here, then you're continuously engaged in a Spiritual Smackdown 24/7. Full of internal conflict, self-sabotage, and held resentments, you will create a life that reflects these beliefs. Exhaustion, confusion, anger, frequent car accidents, relationship breakups, and failed businesses are just some of the ways this struggle can manifest.

Defuse the toxic energy, and delete the debris clouding your thinking by simply remembering that you want to be here. Replace the conflict with the mantra "I wanted to be alive, in this body, in this time. I am open to amazing health and experiences."

If you are struggling in life, take the power back by assuming the power of choice. Remember you chose to be here. And you've had choices every moment since then. We can't always directly and consciously choose what happens, but we can absolutely choose how we respond. If you are starving yourself of experiences that are consistent with your highest purpose, that is akin to choosing to slowly killing yourself. Squandering your passions in exchange for what you 'should' be doing creates an environment rife for disease. You find yourself in conflict with the original choice to be here. You are putting yourself at odds with yourself. This miserable position of having to serve two incompatible masters just makes us end up hating ourselves and our lives.

> *We can't always choose what happens, but we can absolutely choose how we respond.*

Instead of wasting another moment falling down that rabbit hole of despair, start realigning your lifestyle choices with the first choice you made to live in human form. This kind of restructuring has a way of bypassing the ego as we reconnect to our innate wisdom and passion. Tap into that authentic voice within and let go of the ego stories that may have been attacking your business or health success. Most importantly, have courage. If it gives you butterflies that usually means you're doing what you need to do.

If how you want to live is well… that starts by taking stock of your own Giant and envisioning your David.

BE VISIONARY

Can you imagine yourself feeling better? If you've been sick for a long time, this may seem impossible. We could be angry and frustrated year after year for feeling so awful and yet, we can't even imagine ourselves feeling well. We have a vague notion of our desired David-destination, but as to what it looks like in detail, who knows? If Michelangelo hadn't known what David looked like in fantastic detail, he wouldn't have known what to chip away. Similarly, if your own Giant of potential contains wishful thinking instead of specifics, why should you expect it to become something amazing?

Here are some different techniques, tricks and tips to help you harness the power of your inner-eye and envision exactly what you want.

PICTURE YOUR COMPASS

To manifest your David, commit your David-vision to paper in the form of specific goals. Studies have shown that just the act of writing down goals makes it more likely you'll accomplish them. So be sure to aim high, higher even than your doubts and chattering monkey mind is telling you can go. "The greater danger for most of us lies not in setting our aim too high and falling short," Michelangelo once noted, "but in setting our aim too low, and achieving our mark." Setting a worthy mark for yourself means envisioning a shimmering, shining you that has already actualized that vision.

PICTURE YOUR FANTASY ISLAND

When fighting something like illness, it's easy to spend all your thoughts and energy dwelling on your condition. One technique to help lift your energy to a more health-promoting frequency is to imagine a time and a world where you have no illness. Use your imagination lavishly. What do you look like in that world? Maybe you recall a time when you were younger. Others may imagine being in a fantasy world.

If you're tired of thinking about your body as an accumulation of cells that are angry and inflamed, try one of our favorite imaginary worlds where instead of those cells your body is composed of bright yellow smiley faces. Where you have illness or pain, perhaps you see some frown faces. Take time and imagine those frowns turn upside down. See your damaged colon lined with a bunch of happy smiling faces. See your arteries entirely with smiley faces.

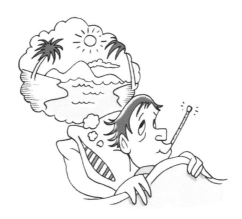

Simplify your thinking about your disease into something more manageable. You know how to change your frown into a smile, so see that happening all over your body. Then, as you go about your day, every time you have a thought about being sick, try to have five more thoughts about your imaginary world of perfect health. There are many ways to dilute a toxic mind and body and giving it new pictures to live by is one of the best.

PICTURE A QUILT

Another way to envision your body's energy is as a lovely protective quilt. When you don't feel well, it begins to tear, usually over diseased areas, but it can be anywhere. Regardless of where any tearing has occurred, imagine mending your quilt with care and attention. As you stitch your energy-quilt back together, you are making it much easier to envision yourself healed. Trust your intuition about where you sense the tears and believe in your power to heal them.

PICTURE FREEDOM

Start to systematically sort through your thoughts, beliefs, fears, joys and experiences. Ask about each: Is this belief/experience aligned with my heart-felt desires? For example, you might ask: Is arguing with my partner all the time unifying my creativity or fracturing it further? Does where I live feed my creativity? Is my job a force for happiness in my life? If you answer yes, then how does it further unify your creative energy? If "no" – why not? When

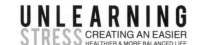

you encounter the self-loathing stories we make up about our lives, the shoulds, woulds, and coulds, decide if this should is really something that helps you feel great. If it doesn't, then the time has come to bid the suggestion goodbye (or adieu or sayonara or Aufweidersehn).

Whatever aspect of your life you put under your belief-magnifying glass, keep looking to see if it helps your authentic spirit shine until you know exactly whether you want to keep it or ditch it. Much like that rose garden you were promised; for it to flourish, there's going to be some pruning involved.

PICTURE IT IN A NEW FRAME

Maybe your job sucks, but it really pays well. It might even pay well enough to fund those (non-free) leisure pursuits you love. Maybe your kids are making you crazy. But you love them more than you could have ever imagined.

In areas of your life that consume huge amounts of your time, attention and energy, perhaps it's time to stop hating it for a moment and think about what it provides: income, love, a unique opportunity to challenge yourself. And maybe, just maybe, it's not the situation that needs to change, it's the way you view it. Sometimes, all you need is to reframe your experience.

PICTURE YOUR INNERSPACE

If you're feeling "stuck" or overwhelmed and not sure where to start visualizing, activate your microcosmic orbit:

> Imagine a bright little sphere of energy about the size of a marble.

> Position it in the center of your chest and then drop it just below the surface of your skin, about ¼ of an inch in, where it will lock into a pathway of energy running down the midline of your body and up the back along the spine, over the top of the head, down the forehead and nose, down the throat, until it connects with the starting point in the chest.

> Start to move the energy ball along the energetic pathway until it completes an entire circuit, however you imagine that.

> If the ball sticks in a particular area and refuses to budge, try gently guiding it with your hands.

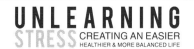

If it will not pass certain areas, veers off the midline or just won't complete the circuit, keep trying to guide the ball on as direct a course as possible as you navigate imbalanced and unsavory areas.

Although this exercise sounds easy, many of my patients who try it often find the opposite; their energy ball stalls at significant blockages or tries to skirt around other areas that are behaving strangely, maybe oozing with creepy energetic sludge, are weirdly cold or piping hot, congested or even dangerously sharp. Whatever you find along the microcosmic orbit, don't judge it.

The harder this meditation is for you, the more you should repeat it daily. Over the course of days, weeks or months, you'll find it gets easier. And when your ball is able to orbit more freely, it's a sign that your Qi is also on the move. This, as you may remember from Chapter #7, Be Active, is the foundation of vibrant health.

PICTURE IT LITERALLY

In this era of CAT scans, MRIs, x-rays, scopes and blood work, we live in an unprecedented time when it comes to being able to see into the body and our innards in all their glory. If you have a colonoscopy that reveals polyps or inflammation, now you know precisely where in the colon to focus your energy and specifically what to focus on in the way of body parts, organs, glands or tissues.

As you target that redness or growth with incredible clarity, you will also be able to focus your energy in a laser-like way seeing it shrink, heal, and the tissues return to their normal size and coloring. Be sure to research or Google what healthy cells are supposed to look like so it's easier for you to visualize yours that way. Seeing what disease looks like and how healthy cells look is knowledge, and knowledge is power – in this case, the cornerstone of your turnaround for two main reasons:

1. You'll know where exactly to focus your healing energies.
2. You'll be able to imagine yourself healed in wildly elaborate detail.

The more detailed and specific your visualizations, the more likely you are to manifest healing. "I want to feel better" is a well-meaning but vague mess of wishful thinking. This specific exercise sends a message to the body and universe that is a clear and focused way to transform your Giant into David.

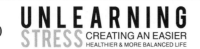

PICTURE A HOLLYWOOD ENDING

If you're sick and go in regularly to your doctor's office, imagine this:

Close your eyes and focus your attention on your breathing. Keep watching your breaths go in and out, in and out, in and out – until you feel some sense of peace.

Now bring to mind to the doctor's office. Populate your mental image with as many details as you can remember:

> Where are you?
>
> What are you wearing?
>
> Does the room have a smell?
>
> Can you see your doctor or nurse?
>
> Any artwork on the walls of the room you're normally in?

Once the scene is set, imagine getting the results of your upcoming scan/blood work/imaging.

Picture your doctor saying:

"Well, we don't really know how it happened, but we can't find any trace of disease anymore. It's amazing and I'm thrilled for you! (This is your visualization…doctors can be thrilled.)

> …or

"Look at this: can you see here on your test results the ulcers are completely healed?"

> …or

"Your heavy metal neutrophil counts are back within the normal range!"

Do this at least three times a day for 15 minutes each. Standing in a line or cooling your heels waiting for an appointment are both perfect times to work on rewriting your history. Reinforce your new and improved version of events. Imagine this experience enough times so that it feels commonplace.

PAINT YOUR ORGANS

According to Chinese medicine, each major energetic organ system is positively influenced by a particular color:

Lungs: white

Heart: red

Spleen: yellow

Liver: green

Kidneys: dark blue/black

To use these associations to heal and strengthen your internal organs, here is a guided-imagery meditation that many of my patients have used with great results.

1. Close your eyes and breathe deeply enough that when you inhale, your abdomen expands and when you breathe out, you feel it pushing the air out of your body and contracting.

2. Once you're comfortably serene, pull out an imaginary paintbrush and starting with your lungs, paint each organ its preferred color, working your way on down to your kidneys. See each paintbrush-stroke as it coats an organ. What other details can you infuse your image with? Remember: it is the details that are the secret to succeeding with guided meditations.

3. As you're painting each organ, observe how it responds to its color. Is it particularly receptive to it? Does it "refuse" to take the color on your brush? Whatever the reaction, be sure not to judge it – just observe as you paint how each organ reacts. These reactions are your body's way of giving you vital information about yourself. Also, the act of painting starts to correct energetic imbalances which will enable damaged cells to heal.

4. After you've done a first pass of painting all your organs, step back and admire your handiwork. Uh oh, is that a spot without color over there? Go back and try again to see if the organ is now more receptive. Take a look at how all the colors are interacting with each other. Are they staying clearly defined or running together? Again, no judging.

UNLEARNING STRESS CREATING AN EASIER HEALTHIER & MORE BALANCED LIFE

5. Now visualize yourself standing under a waterfall. The water first hits the top of your head and then enters it, washing over your freshly-painted organs and splish-splashing away the colors along with any imbalances and disease. Watch as the impurities wash out the bottom of your feet and return to the earth. Savor the sensation that your organs are now functioning freely and your balance has been restored. Open your eyes, take a deep breath, and take another moment to enjoy how you feel.

ADD SOME SPICE

WATCH: some documentaries about the maestro for inspiration, including *Michelangelo: Self Portrait* (2010) – narrated in the artist's own words and shot by an Oscar-winning director on location in Italy; *Michelangelo: Captured in Stone* (2011); *Michelangelo: Artist and Man* A&E Biography (2004).

READ: Any or all of these will reinforce your cooking skills with this chapter: *The Power of Visualization: Meditation Secrets that Matter Most* by Sri Vishwanath; *Return to the Sacred* by Jonathan Ellerby; *Reprogram Your Subconscious: Use the Power of Your Mind to Get Everything You Want* by Kelly Wallace; *Heal Your Mind, Rewire Your Brain: Applying the Exciting New Science of Brain Synchrony for Creativity, Peace and Presence* by Patt Lind-Kyle, MA

CREATE: your own picture of what you want with a Vision Board. Here are some ways to "do" one (or a bunch): *Visioning: Ten Steps to Designing the Life of Your Dreams; The Complete Vision Board Kit: Using the Power of Intention and Visualization to Achieve Your Dreams*

LISTEN: *The Angel Inside: Michelangelo's Secrets For Following Your Passion and Finding the Work You Love* (Audiobook; 2007) When a young boy once asked the artist why he was working so hard on The Giant, he replied, "Young man, there is an angel inside this rock, and I am setting him free." What angels are inside you, just waiting to be set free?

ADVANCE: your mindset by bypassing your monkey-mind gatekeeper. *Inner Talk's (www.innertalk.com)* award-winning subliminal programs go around the resistant part of your mind to appeal to the subconscious and help you change your internal chatter.

CHANNEL: your inner Michelangelo with *The Michelangelo Method: Release Your Inner Masterpiece and Create an Extraordinary Life* by Kenneth Schuman. A mix of examples from the artist's life, case studies from life-coaching and exercises.

SUMMARY

Chapter 8: Be Visionary

- Can you imagine yourself feeling better? Great success, health, businesses, houses, and artwork often start from being able to see the finished product before anyone else. See yourself feeling better, even if it demands every bit of your imagination.

- Trust that you have more control than you realize to create the life you want. Be an active participant in dreaming up the world, health, and success you want.

- If you are sick, imagine every cell in your body being healthy. Focus on the diseased areas and reprogram your body with positive imagery specifically shrinking and destroying diseased cells and replacing them with healthy new ones. Create the blueprint for your body, mind, and spirit to follow.

FOOD FOR THOUGHT FOR CHAPTER 8

Is it easy or difficult to envision perfect and total health for you? If it is difficult, is there someone you admire that has the attributes you want in your life? Picture that person in great detail and then see their face as yours. Make it your own.

If you believe (maybe just for a second) the suggestion that you chose to be born, why do you think you did? Why did you choose your parents? Why might you have chosen your hometown or to be in a family with your siblings? Why during this time period? Can you weave these feelings into your vision for your life?

Take your vision for your life and hold it up against everything that is currently in your life, your entire day to day interactions. Does this person/place/thing that you are interacting with support or detract from your vision for life? If it detracts, why do you keep it in your energy space? Is there something else you can do with your perception of it or with its actual presence in your life? Can you turn your relationship with this person/place/thing into one that is supportive and nurturing of your vision? How will you start that process?

Chapter # 9 : Be Spontaneous

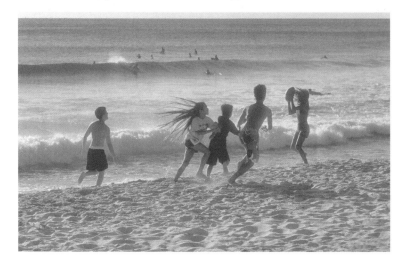

"Once we believe in ourselves, we can risk curiosity, wonder, spontaneous delight, or any experience that reveals the human spirit."

— e.e. cummings

A patient of mine suffered fibromyalgia. When she sensed a flare-up looming, she threw all her attention and energy, every thought and action, into trying to control the symptoms of the intense pain to keep her suffering to a minimum. This wasn't working, which is why she ended up in my office. Instead, I gently suggested she simply let a flare up happen, sit with it through its progressions and instead of fighting it, observe it. Needless to say, she initially found the suggestion horrifying.

Having always fought her symptoms, she was afraid of what it meant to not fight. But as she tested this new approach, not only did her energy downshift and become much calmer and far less reactive, but surprisingly – for her – her flare-ups became much shorter.

Instead of lasting days or weeks, the flare ups started to come and go in a matter of hours or minutes. By replacing her fear with alert watchfulness, she did something remarkable: she no longer approached her condition having already made up her mind about what to expect based on past experiences.

UNLEARNING STRESS CREATING AN EASIER HEALTHIER & MORE BALANCED LIFE

JAMES ROHR, L.Ac

By removing her assumptions and foregone conclusions, she created new energetic circuits that included new possibilities: that her flare-ups could change for the better and with much less work, tension and stress on her part. This discovery, in turn, prompted her to rethink how she dealt with adversity in general. Without the baggage of flare-up expectations, she became receptive not only to alternative ways of being with her flare-ups, but in the rest of her life.

> *"Empty your mind, be formless, shapeless – like water.*
>
> *Now you put water into a cup, it becomes the cup.*
>
> *You put water into a bottle, it becomes the bottle.*
>
> *You put it in a teapot, it becomes the teapot.*
>
> *Now water can flow or it can crash. Be water my friend."*
>
> *- Bruce Lee*

Putting into practice what we've been discussing in the various chapters creates fertile ground for healing. Once you've sowed the seeds, kept the weeds at bay, watered and protected your emotional garden, your job is simply to wait.

But watchfully wait. Great health, miraculous recovery, and/or enlightenment could happen this very moment. Are you paying attention? If your head is elsewhere, planning, doing, hoping, expecting, demanding, and trying to control the future, you're missing what is happening right now. "When you're busy making other plans," the saying goes, "life is what happens."

Over the years, I have been amazed at how people try to control their recovery from illness. They hope and pray for a miracle, and then when presented with various healing options, they say things like, "oh no, that's not for me. I don't believe in it. I'm waiting for this other way to work out." When the universe responds to our energy and prayers, we have to be paying attention or else we might miss it. How many times do you have to hear about an option before acting upon it?

If you're busy planning your future recovery, then you might be cutting off the flow of possibilities happening in this very moment. While great health happens, the when and where are not always up to you. What is up to you is the choice to remain in the now.

Remember: to succeed in healing, to attain that lovely grace of feeling whole, you have to be in it – the moment.

Your body is constantly changing. Each moment you are a new version of you, uniquely interacting with your environment. The cells and signals those cells send to the brain are constantly changing. Your pain or sufferings, no matter how familiar they feel, are triggered by a new set of cells and energy. You've responded to different emotional, mental, and environmental stimuli. Treating each moment as a unique entity means we can break free from the stories of the past and all the expected outcomes. When we live in the moment, without attachment, we start to become attuned to those moments of divine grace. When our Qi is flowing freely, then great health may be awaiting us right now, in this moment, spontaneously.

Spontaneously shifting energy happens even if you suffer chronic pain or illness; at times, the symptoms will ease or vanish, even fleetingly. Do you recognize these moments and respond by saying "thank you"? Gratitude begets more good things, so as you welcome each moment of great health, you create the potential for still more to arrive. At any moment. And when each arrives, allow yourself the joy of being delighted. For a chronically ill person, spontaneity means being present, and allowing for the possibility that in this moment, your energy may be infused with the exact stimulus you've needed to feel better. Will you be aware enough to notice it? Can you imagine that in this next moment you may have the perfect alignment of mind/body/spirit for you to have total health?

Spontaneity is the exact opposite of what we want from things with buttons. We've been using these techniques to stop being robotic and start being freely human. Spontaneity is what will prevent that usual tidal wave of toxic thoughts from gaining momentum and crashing violently about you, drowning you in an emotional flood of fear, anger and self-pity.

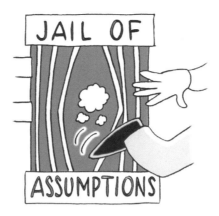

Good thing that Now is such an amazing place to be. As you greet each moment spontaneously, you enter a special state of being unshackled by the confines of the past. Thomas Edison is said to have failed at least a gazillion times[115] to create the light bulb he had envisioned. However, instead of allowing himself the luxury of retreating into self-recrimination or doubt, he focused on the fact that he now knew yet another way not to make a light bulb. This meant the correct way was still awaiting him. The takeaway is that just because something hasn't been done before doesn't mean it's not possible. Strong precedent is past history, nothing more. And you can think the same things as "everyone else" or you can start to believe in possibilities. The power of possibilities becomes apparent when you stay in the now, greeting each new moment spontaneously. That 'now' contains infinite possibility, including instantaneous healing.

We are so much more capable than we tend to believe. Why do we insist on limiting ourselves to living in a paradigm enshrouded by what "everyone else" believes? Instead of groping about in the pre-Edison dark and calling that "your life", why not set your preconceived ideas aside and increase your capacity for limitless opportunity from its current one-gallon size to two or five … or who knows.

OBSERVE AND EXPERIENCE

Yep, back to some of our meditation techniques now! One of the ways to train your spontaneity muscles is by working on being really observant. Spend at least 60 seconds looking at and listening to your environment. When you hear a noise, simply listen without deciding what you think is causing the sound. Even though we've done this one before, resist the temptation to think you know it. Try it again. Instead of making associations as to what is creating the sound, just notice the sound of the siren, the changes in loudness as it nears and departs. Simply experience.

LEARN TO SEE

Take a close look at a white wall in your living space. You'll start to notice you actually see very little true-white color. There are shadows and various shades of yellow, grays, ambers and others. Painting classes are great for this exercise because you learn how to really see, especially colors. But our minds make assumptions because we think we know things. Cease the knowing and just observe. This practice is one of the best to get out of your incessant mental chatter and into your sense organs. If we are to fully enjoy this life, let's use all of our senses to the fullest. But so long as we think we know everything, we stop paying attention and stop taking in new information.

LIFESTYLE YOURSELF BETTER

Mind, spirit and body are intimately connected, inseparable really, so if you mistreat the one, you can't expect to maximize the potential of the others. A great place to start expanding your capacity for spontaneous awesomeness is with healthy lifestyle choices, like not smoking, drinking like a fish or eating too much junk. Ask yourself:

> Have I aligned my mind/body/spirit to be in the best possible place to manifest the energetic transformation I've been visualizing?
>
> Am I open to the possibility?
>
> Would I recognize it if it happened right now or am I too busy complaining or worrying?

PLAN AHEAD

The sudden appearance of flowers at the start of spring belies the tremendous movement and growth beneath in the soil that lead to the season's first blooms. Similarly, a healing can appear instantaneous, but in fact it rests on a firm foundation of good self-care that encompasses all aspects of yourself, from eating right to sitting in meditation to breaking through your mental stumbling blocks.

ADD SOME SPICE

MOVE LIKE A CHA CHA CHAMP: *The Art of Expressing the Human Body* by Bruce Lee. The martial arts movie star was also an insightful philosopher, which his physical training reflected. Like water, he adapted and changed, never standing still. Pair it with *Striking Thoughts: Bruce Lee's Wisdom for Daily Living*, part of the excellent Bruce Lee Library series. (Lee could also dance, winning the Hong Kong Cha Cha Championship in 1958 when he was 18.[116])

SEE LIKE AN ARTIST: Learn to see the world beyond what you assumed or expected to be there. The world we live in continually reinforces left-brain dominance over our experiences, filtering everything through a haze of "I thought this's" and "I assumed that's". *Drawing on the Right Side of the Brain: the Definitive 4th Edition* (2012) by Betty Edwards is a clever book that not only teaches you how to trick your left hemisphere into relinquishing control for a moment, allowing you to surprise yourself at what you can actually draw, but start to perceive more of the connectedness in the world. A gem!

HEAL LIKE YOU MEAN IT: *Spontaneous Healing: How to Discover and Enhance: Your Body's Natural Ability to Maintain and Heal Itself* by Andrew Weil, M.D. From the placebo effect, to inexplicable remissions to even the commonplace repair of wounds, your body is primed to heal itself. *The Spontaneous Healing of Belief: Shattering the Paradigm of False Limits* by Gregg Braden

SUMMARY

Chapter 9: Be Spontaneous

- Every moment you witness in your lifetime is unique. The mistake is to think that things are always the same and never change. A cornerstone of deep healing is recognizing the unique potential that exists in every new moment.

- Being spontaneous allows you to break from the robotic, unconscious way of being into a more engaged and enlightened place.

- A great way to retrain your focus on the moment is to take up painting or photography classes. Discover a new way to see the world and use this same skill to transform your health and life.

FOOD FOR THOUGHT FOR CHAPTER 9

What things/people/events do you allow to take you out of the moment?

Has this list changed or is it different from the very first list you made of your fight or flight triggers in Chapter 2?

If the same things keep coming up, how do you think that is impacting your shift to greater wellness?

If time, energy, money, and consequence were of no concern, what would you like to do with your life?

Chapter # 10 : Be Limitless

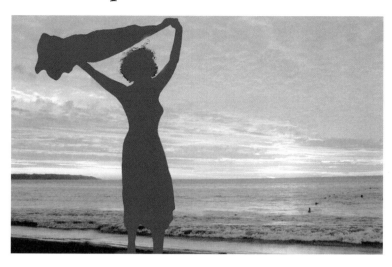

The artist's world is limitless. It can be found anywhere, far from where he lives or a few feet away. It is always on his doorstep.

— Paul Strand

Once you start living your life from moment to moment, spontaneously, you start to relinquish the need to predetermine the outcome of whatever chapter of your own personal story you're currently in. Life is a mystery. A Mystery School, actually, with a curriculum devoted 100% to your spiritual development here in your human form. Classes are structured around the challenges you face, and those challenges manifest because of what you need to grow and learn. It seems to me that your higher spiritual self chose your foundation in advance of your being born, including your parents, where you would be born and when.

"Ever since your birth, it [your higher self] has been orchestrating ALL the events and people in your life to perfectly present you with all the challenges and lessons you most need in order to develop yourself," notes Dr. Asoka Selvarajah, an author and researcher in the field of Esoteric Spirituality. "From this perspective, nothing happens in your life by chance. Everything has meaning. There are no accidents."[117]

So if you're facing a situation you find to be quite challenging, I say 'Congratulations!' The tougher the test in the School of Life, the higher your status. It means you're one high-ranking ninja.

And many of your fellow spiritual ninjas – and maybe you as well – are all in the midst of one particularly tough test: a scary prognosis. The diagnosis is an umbrella which encompasses the possible progression of symptoms, their intensity and the likelihood of recovery – and based on these expectations, determines the standard of care and interventions, whether that is surgery, medication, diet, exercise. Without the framework of a diagnosis, each illness would be seen as completely new and unpredictable, meaning healthcare providers would have to "reinvent the wheel" each time.

With a standard diagnostic procedure, people are grouped together based on signs and symptoms, constitution or pattern. This makes it much easier to develop a standard of care and then communicate that assessment to others in the business quickly, conveniently and (hopefully) accurately. Basically, a diagnosis is simply a language that healthcare practitioners use to communicate with each other quickly and easily – i.e. a shorthand.

> *Stressed spelled backwards is*
>
> *D-E-S-S-E-R-T-S. Coincidence?*
>
> *I think not.*
>
> *—Anonymous*

The trouble is, the shorthand is often too "short" for the complexity of the situation. The combination of a relatively new medicine, coupled with the cold and foreign sounding –itis and –omas, this western medicine shorthand can really suck. Even when trying to be more broad and poetic, the English language leaves a lot to be desired: "The English language is not designed for this conversation," points out Gregg Braden, best-selling author of *The God Code* and *The Divine Matrix*. "In Sanskrit there is one word that means the energy body of the human, for example. It's prana. In English, there is no single word for prana, so we have to take other words and put them together: energy body, or electrical magnetic field, or something like that."[118]

UNLEARNING STRESS CREATING AN EASIER HEALTHIER & MORE BALANCED LIFE

A diagnosis is no different: while the attempt to describe the situation is admirable, we need to be careful to assign it too much power or importance. Unfortunately, though, when most of us are diagnosed with something scary. "The doctor said so" factor kicks in, giving the diagnosis more weight than it may deserve.[119] A good doctor is just doing their job within the current paradigm of practice, but that doesn't make whatever they say "so". It's just another perspective. Never forget that. All a diagnosis really is is a different lens with which to see yourself.

Compare two scenarios. A sick patient walks into the doctor's office and…

… gets the good prognosis they yearn for. "If other people have healed, surely I have a chance," s/he thinks. "Ahh, at least "they" know what I have, it's [INSERT NAME OF CONDITION] and I'm not alone in this. There are others who have experienced this and when they received the standard treatment for these signs and symptoms, it worked for them!" Here, the diagnosis is accurate and the patient responds favorably, so it's a part of an efficient and effective treatment process.

… after receiving what s/he thinks is bad news, immediately starts scanning the pamphlet the doctor gave them, looking for the worst-case scenario (much like the patient who becomes hyperaware of all the side-effect warnings that accompany a prescription drug, steadfastly believing they will get most – if not all – of the dreaded side-effects). Fear floods their psyche and suddenly,

> *'Believe nothing, no matter where you read it,*
>
> *or who said it, no matter if I have said it,*
>
> *unless it agrees with your own reason*
>
> *and your own common sense.'*
>
> *Buddha*

the same apparent predictability that gave the patient in the first scenario peace of mind has the opposite effect and becomes a major hurdle to overcome in healing. Healing, as you know by now, is very difficult within an environment of fear.

The bad news? The impersonal-shorthand of a diagnosis does not take into account your subtle differences. The good news? The impersonal-shorthand of a diagnosis does not take into account your subtle differences. The peculiarities of who you are might be precisely what enable you to defy your diagnosis and to heal. Why? Because just by being alive and conscious, you are directly affecting the outcome of the world around you. Physicists have found that at the quantum level of the world, we are not onlookers but participants playing the prime role in creating our lives.

"In a participatory universe," continues Braden, "you and I are part of the equation. We are both creating the events of our lives, as well as the experiencers of what we create…In other words, we are like artists expressing our deepest passions, fears, dreams and desires through the living essence of a mysterious quantum canvas."[120] Which means that if you deem a diagnosis to be a death sentence, it is. If you want to heal, you must be spontaneous and in the moment. Expecting negative outcomes or limiting your possibility to heal, even if no one else in the history of the world has overcome the illness you have, means that you expect to remain sick.

Fortunately, research has shown we have a head start when it comes to our expectations because we are mostly all hard-wired to be optimists.

Our natural drive is to explore and create, to enjoy the world and frolic in it. And when anything happens to deter us from that natural optimism, such as a diagnosis of "You have this disease and you will always have it…" it can smush hope altogether. But don't let it!

"Hope, whether internally generated, or coming from an outside source, enables people to embrace their goals and stay committed to moving toward them," explains Tali Sharot, Ph.D. in psychology and neuro-science from New York University, and author of *The Optimism Bias*. "This behavior will eventually make the goal more likely to become a reality."

Put differently, even "false" hope is better than no hope because feeling hopeless can turn you into a "defensive" pessimist[121] and pessimists tend to fare less well in life, including illness. "Low expectations do not diminish the pain of failure," continues Sharot. "Not only do negative expectations lead to

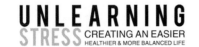

worse results; they also fail to protect us from negative emotions when unwanted outcomes occur."

What are your limitations to healing? Make a list. Is it money? Time? Lack of knowledge? Bad diagnosis? Bad doctors? Botched treatments? Side effects of medications? Tired of being tired? Undoubtedly, this can become a very long list. Take your time. We're not going anywhere. Hopefully, as you've been following the previous lessons, this list is not as long as it would've been at the start.

Now, tear up the list. All of those things may have been true in your past. But they need not apply now. This moment is full of new breath, new life, and new energy. Your experience of yourself and this moment can entirely change the trajectory you were on. Let go of the limitations and be thankful that this moment may have the enlightenment you've been hoping for.

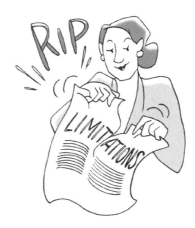

But don't believe me. Begin to concentrate your energy in a way to manifest your true potential. As you've been doing over the entire 'year' of this book, you now have the wherewithal to focus your energy more precisely. Chapter 8, Be Visionary, is one of the most important. We must see the change in great detail. Cultivating your meditation skills in Chapter 3, Be Seated, also helps to clear away the clutter of our energy field akin to cleaning your windshield so you can see things more clearly. The Chinese medicine martial art of Qi Gong has been my favorite form of self-healing[122].

As we saw in Chapter 8, rather than working toward being healed, feel – really feel – that you have been healed and live from that place of having

UNLEARNING
STRESS CREATING AN EASIER
HEALTHIER & MORE BALANCED LIFE

arrived. Stop asking to be healed or praying for change. Assume the change or healing has already happened and capitalize on that energy. Be Grateful (Chapter 5) for the gift of the healing that has already happened. While our little reptilian brain may fight our sense of non-linear time, he'll soon be drowned out in all the feel-good energy that your body creates as it swims in the sea of positive imagery.

Feeling total health isn't something I can teach you – not me, not Buddha, not your favorite preacher or spiritual teacher. Total health, emotional freedom and incredible health, must be directly experienced by you. You define what total health means to you and it will be up to you to manifest it, one moment after another. "I have experience," Joseph Campbell once said. "I don't need faith." Nor do you. Have no faith in anything I say or write. Rather, work the techniques in this book for yourself and when you start feeling better, build on that. When you don't believe any of the limits other people put on your capabilities, then anything is possible. And when anything is possible, health is possible. Which means you have every reason in the world (you're creating) to be optimistic and limitless.

ADD SOME SPICE

READ: *Secrets of the Lost Mode of Prayer: The Hidden Power of Beauty, Blessings, Wisdom and Hurt* by Gregg Braden; *The Emotion Code* by Bradley Nelson (ways to rid yourself of unwanted emotional baggage keeping you back); *Frequency: The Power of Personal Vibration* by Penney Peirce (keep your energy vibrating groovily); *Energy Medicine: Balancing Your Body's Energies for Optimal Health, Joy and Vitality* by Donna Eden *The Optimism Bias* by Tali Sharot.

WATCH: *The Science of Healing* with Dr. Esther Sternberg; *The Knowledge of Healing* featuring the Dalai Lama; *BreakThrough: A Conscious Documentary; Beyond Belief; Three Magic Words, The Thought Exchange – a Practical Method of Moving Beyond Positive Thinking.*

EMOTE: in a more healthy way. Emotions start with the physical, so elevate yours to a healthier wavelength with body-focus and breathing techniques as outlined in *Quantum Touch: The Power to Heal* by Richard Gordon.

LEARN: more about the Essenes with *Creating Peace by Being Peace: the Essene Sevenfold Path* by Gabriel Cousens, MD.

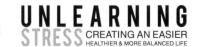

CREATE: a healthier you by walking the walk. These approaches will help you practice what we've been preaching: *Revive: Stop Feeling Spent and Start Living Again* by Frank Lipman, M.D. and *The Source: Unleash Your Natural Energy, Power Up Your Health and Feel 10 Years Younger* by Woodson Merrell, M.D. Both are medical doctors with a holistic outlook.

SUMMARY

Chapter 10: Be Limitless

- The time has come to blow the doors open to what you think is possible. Expand your horizons. Give yourself permission to feel great. Don't let anyone tell you what is not possible.

- A diagnosis is just another way of viewing the world. It is another perspective to ascertain part of how you are feeling. You are more than your diagnosis.

- The peculiarities of who you are may be precisely what allow you to heal, even if no one else has healed from this particular disease or imbalance before you.

FOOD FOR THOUGHT FOR CHAPTER 10

Are you hopeful for a full recovery? If not, why not? Do you believe other people's suggestions about what they believe are or are not possible for you? Do they have an idea of what should or should not be happening?

What if you never had a diagnosis? Would your relationship be different with your body?

What are some other places in your life where other people's suggestions and ideas about your life are getting in your way? Make a list of all the suggestions that may still be lying in wait in the recesses of your mind.

Can you be grateful for everyone and everything found on that list? Can you move beyond those suggestions to sing your song, to sound your own barbaric yawp across the world?

If you had one message you can share with the world, one thing that everyone would hear and know that it came from you, what would it be?

 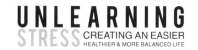

Study Guide

Chapter 1: Be Present

- Why is something as simple as breathing the first, and most important, chapter?
- How does your breathing change when you are stressed out?
- How many breaths does a qi gong practice recommend you have per minute?
- When is the best time to do diaphragmatic breathing?

Chapter 2: Be Calm

- What are the names of the two nervous systems?
- Which one is primarily active during rest and relaxation?
- How can something that used to be so helpful (the fight/flight response) now be causing so much damage?
- What is the difference between imagined and real threats to your well-being?
- What is the connection between the fight/flight response and your breathing?

Chapter 3: Be Seated

- Is the initial function of meditation to clear your mind?
- Do you have to sit in front of a candle in a dark room in order to meditate?
- What is the greatest gift of mindfulness practice?
- Do you have any control over your reactions to stress?
- According to recent studies, list four of the benefits of meditation and mindfulness?

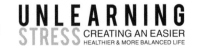

Chapter 4: Be Nourished

- How does diet seem to affect chronic illness?
- How does processed food affect the bacteria in the gut?
- Is fat good for you? What are ideal sources of fat?
- Why is bone broth healthy?
- What are the health benefits of fermented foods?
- Why are gluten and other whole grains a concern?

Chapter 5: Be Grateful

- What is the relationship between the energy of a 'thank-you' and the nervous systems in the body?
- Why do I suggest being thankful for everything in life, even for hard times and illness?
- Why are unmet expectations so dangerous?
- Why is forgiveness so important to healing?
- What are three areas in your life that could benefit from forgiveness and a little extra gratitude?

Chapter 6: Be Connected

- What are the dangers of loneliness?
- What are some of the benefits of shifting from a vertical hierarchy to a horizontal symbiotic relationship with your environment?
- Explain three ways you can increase your feeling of being connected and in good relationships.
- What is the Chinese concept of Jing/Essence?
- What is the effect of sex on the Jing?

Chapter 7: Be Active

- What is the relationship between yin, yang, qi and movement?
- What are the two key ways that exercise helps the body?
- What are two types of neuro-motor exercise conditioning?

Chapter 8: Be Visionary

- Why is the David story so important?
- What is the connection between imagination and healing?
- What is the microcosmic orbit and how do you use it to move your energy?

Chapter 9: Be Spontaneous

- What are some of the benefits of being in the moment?
- What does painting a picture have to do with being spontaneous in the moment?
- How does being spontaneous affect the should, would, and could?

Chapter 10: Be Limitless

- What is a diagnosis?
- How does being a unique human being impact your disease?
- What is the danger of negative emotions?

UNLEARNING STRESS CREATING AN EASIER HEALTHIER & MORE BALANCED LIFE

JAMES ROHR, L.Ac

Q and A with James Rohr, Acupuncture Physician

What is the main message you hope people take-away from reading *Unlearning Stress?*

I hope people take away from this book ideas, tools, and resources to feel more alive, more energized, and more free. We do this by calling our attention to our internal behavior and how we relate to our outside world with our food, thoughts, relationships, and spiritual health.

What inspired the book?

This book is the first published material from stuff that I began writing in 2004 when I was in my mid-twenties. I had been feeling the inclination to write, so I decided to sit down one day and see what I had to say. For about a year and a half, I would write as much as possible. I cut back my clinical hours to devote myself to writing. It was a very inspired time. Even today, when I look back at the 300 pages that composed the initial draft of my early musings, some sections feel like they were written by someone else. I clearly remember the little alcove in Chicago where I did most of the writing. It was as if there was a faucet of energy above my head. When I sat down, I opened up the faucet, and let my fingers type away. When I was able to keep my monkey mind quiet, the insights were beautiful.

After being recruited in 2008 to Miami Beach to be the head acupuncturist for Canyon Ranch's new location in Miami Beach, I shifted my focus from writing to building the clinical practice there. A few years later, I felt the itch to write again. This book, *Unlearning Stress*, is the first of several I have planned that synthesizes my early material with the changing needs of the modern patient. I am very proud of how this book has turned out and I hope people will find it helpful to begin to overcome their imbalances and ultimately feel freer in their lives.

Why did you call it *Unlearning Stress?*

This book turned out to be a collection of things that I find myself saying over and over again in my clinic and lectures. It's been said that we are human beings and yet most people these days are human doings. We are quickly forgetting how to simply be us: authentic, inspired, and free. Consumed

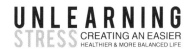

with trying be how other people want you to be or how you think should be is not being 'healthy' or truly alive. Following the steps in the book will help people to actualize the fullness of their capabilities as a human being and the freedom that is inherent in this thing we call life.

What sorts of things do you see in your practice?

I treat a wide variety of issues in my practice. Stress related disorders is what I refer to a wide variety illnesses often including insomnia, low energy, chronic fatigue, headaches, digestive upset, and chronic pain. I see men's and women's health concerns as well as lots of sports and orthopedic medicine.

Sections of this book grow directly from my years of working with people on meditation. I wanted to have one resource that makes the case for why mindfulness is important and offers techniques and theories to get that process started. I am continually amazed at how easy it is for us to behave like hamsters in a cage running in the wheel all day long. Let's step off that wheel and take a deep breath, look around, and fill up with gratitude at being alive in this playground that is Earth.

So much illness is due to poor diet and poor stress management skills. We could talk about herbs, medications, and supplements for thousands of pages (believe me, I spent a long time in school learning this stuff), but if you are eating toxic food, thinking toxic thoughts, and generally not striving to be conscious, there is only so much wellness that can be attained. Symptom-free is not the same as being healthy. True wealth in wellness comes from being fully conscious of the moment.

What authors do you like and do you have any suggested reading?

In the 'self-help' genre, two books were formative in my development as a healer: Carolyn Myss' *Anatomy of the Spirit* and Barbara Ann Brennan's *Hands of Light*. Of course, it is tough to linger in the alternative health realm without reading at least one of Carlos Castaneda's books. *The Teachings of Don Juan* was a great read for my teenage mind. My 'spiritual awakening' directly coincided with my discovering a love for poetry. Walt Whitman's exuberant writings and respect for the earth continue to remind me of the love that permeates all life. Gary Snyder continues this theme and more recently Billy Collins is always enjoyable for me.

Siddhartha by Hesse was also incredible as is *Full Catastrophe Living* by Jon Kabat-Zinn. More recently, books that have inspired me or moved me in some way include *The Road* by Cormac McCarthy, *The Talent Code* by Daniel Coyle, and Jack Hawley's version of *the Bhagavad Gita*. Of course, the list wouldn't be complete without mentioning my earliest and most formative literary influence: *Calvin and Hobbes* by Watterson....all collections.

What was your experience at Stanford like?

My time at Stanford was incredible. There's a quote I've heard that says "If you're the smartest person in the room, you're in the wrong room!" Let's just say I never had to leave a room at Stanford (after all, it took me two tries to get accepted. I did my freshman year at the University of Notre Dame and transferred to Stanford for my sophomore year). Being surrounded by brilliant people is definitely the way to go. I was honored to be considered a peer.

Beyond the student body, the institutional support for undergraduate research is what defined my Stanford academic experience. I was able to acquire funding to travel to the Peruvian jungle for research on eco-tourism, to Sicily for an archaeological dig, and then back to Peru to spend a summer in the highlands doing archaeological research.

Back on campus, I lived in a cooperative house where we cooked and cleaned for ourselves. 40 students living in one house with co-ed bathrooms and showers! The Theta Chi co-operative house celebrated the pursuit of your passion. We were pretty self-determined, and it was there that I felt the support to go on and pursue Chinese medicine. If I had lived anywhere else, I might not have been brave enough to see this career thru.

What do the readers need to know?

Everything happens in the moment. That is all that matters. What happened yesterday, when you were young, or in past lives does not have the power we think it does. The power resides in committing to the moment and knowing that you have the power to alter your perception of the moment, every day, and every moment, forever. When it comes to your health, when we think we know how something works or what will or won't happen, especially just

UNLEARNING STRESS CREATING AN EASIER HEALTHIER & MORE BALANCED LIFE

because someone else says that will happen, we have to be vigilant in seeing how each moment has its own potential where anything is possible.

There are a lot of self-help books out there now. How is yours different?

There are a lot of self-help books, but very few have been written in English intended for the general audience by a Chinese medicine practitioner. Chinese medicine has an incredible array of treatments developed over the last 5,000 years. I have taken some of my favorite insights from Chinese medicine and woven them into very practical, easy-to-implement suggestions for people to start living their best life. While this book doesn't include much by way of direct advice from Chinese medicine, the overall themes and suggestions should be familiar to anyone who has studied the medicine or Eastern philosophies.

What is your favorite section in the book?

I am particularly fond of *Be Grateful*. Gratitude is so powerful and needs to be the default setting for our lives. No matter if you're angry, sad, alone, joyous, celebrating, in pain or disease free, life on earth is an incredible ride, so let's be thankful for it. Thank you for my anger. Thank you for my pain. I don't know exactly who the 'you' is that we're thanking, but maybe it is the cosmic water that we all unwittingly swim in. Or maybe it's your parents and grandparents and their relatives. Think about the entire string of events that have conspired over the course of history to make this exact moment happen for you! Absolutely incredible.

There's a visualization that I'll use sometimes at the end of my qi gong classes that I'll share here. Imagine standing behind you are your parents. And imagine behind them are their parents. And behind them are your great grandparents. Imagine all of your relatives and ancestors lining up behind you for as far as you can imagine. Feel the enormity of the moment that you are experiencing all because they lived before you. This is absolutely amazing. Now, imagine yourself turning around to face them. See the crowd of your family tree. And now, slightly bow your head and say thank you to all your relations.

Where do I start with these changes?

Start now, with this very moment. But throughout the process, be kind and understanding with yourself. Replacing one focus of an addiction to another isn't helpful. If the self-talk is shaming and overly-critical, there is no amount of exercise that can outrace an overly critical mind. Being awake and alert is one of the hardest and the simplest things to do. Each moment is infused with so much energy that all we have to do is allow ourselves to breathe it in. We don't have to lift it, sculpt it, create it, or muscle it to happen. We just have to get out of our own way. For those of us who have no idea how we are in our own way, this awakening process can be difficult. Yet, there is nothing more rewarding for me than becoming aware.

What is Oriental medicine school?

I enrolled in Chinese medicine school directly after graduating from Stanford. The degree is a Master's of Science, but unlike most masters programs that are one or two years, this program is four years. I went to a fantastic school called Pacific College of Oriental Medicine. With over 3500 hours of training, the coursework includes the western stuff: physiology, pathophysiology, pharmacology, anatomy, chemistry, and orthopedic and neurological assessment; the eastern stuff: acupuncture point location, needling techniques, individual herbs, herbal formulas, theory, theory, and more theory. The program also includes clinical rotations, qi gong, tai chi, and bodywork classes. The program is robust and not for the faint of heart. There is so much material out there that it could take many lifetimes to master it.

Any personal discoveries for you while studying Chinese medicine?

One of the things I quickly realized in Chinese medicine school is that people are suffering. They are suffering with ailments that are often easily treated by things other than traditional western medicine. If they can get out of their own limiting beliefs and incorporate other treatment options, their relationship to their chronic conditions would most likely change. It is my hopes that as people read this book and realize that it is full of good, practical information, they will be more inclined to follow up with their local acupuncturist for more direct care if that is needed.

UNLEARNING STRESS CREATING AN EASIER HEALTHIER & MORE BALANCED LIFE

Talk about your first major job after you graduated from Chinese medicine school. You were part of the integrative medicine at a major hospital system in the Chicago area. This was one of the earliest integrative medicine centers of its kind.

Working in affiliation with a hospital in the Midwest was interesting because I saw firsthand people's reluctance to try something new. There is a certain type of person who is more comfortable sticking within their hospital system, even though we were an out-patient facility. I tended to see people who were very sick: cancer, Parkinson's, fibromyalgia, chronic pain, etc. People would come in saying, "I don't really want to be here, but I'm out of options. I've tried everything else and you're my last hope to feel better." I remember thinking, "Wow. What a responsibility!"

Eventually, I realized that for most of these people, they hadn't actually tried everything. They may have exhausted reasonable western conventional medicine options, but an entire world of 'alternative' or 'complementary' treatments was still untapped. This book is designed to fill in some of those gaps to introduce them to a variety of techniques and resources that can complement their work with a licensed healthcare provider.

First and foremost, though, I had to educate these patients that the only one that was going to get them feeling better was themselves. Health is a reflection of our internal energy as it relates and interacts with our external environment. If you're inclined to include this next phase, I would also say that health is a reflection of our internal energy as it relates and interacts with the Divine. They didn't 'need' me to get them feeling better. All I can do is give the body a little bit of direction, or give their mind some new ideas to help shift their energy, but they were the ones who would do the work. If they returned to a toxic world, there's not much I can do. If their thoughts were limiting and toxic, there's only so much health that could happen. We have to reclaim the power we've surrendered to our doctor's and/or diagnoses, and recognize that the grace that makes us uniquely us is what is going to initiate and maintain our healing.

You created the first mobile application for Chinese medicine tongue diagnosis called Tungz!. Talk a bit about that.

I've been giving lectures on tongue assessment for many years now, and I thought the subject matter would lend itself to a nice app. I'm a big fan of technology and education, so this app is a natural combination of those two interests. The app has pictures of tongues and explains the meanings of them. The most important thing is for people to realize what a 'healthy' tongue looks like and the notice their own. If it doesn't look like the healthy one, then it is time to start working on your energy level to start feeling better. As you begin to improve the quality and flow of your Qi, your tongue will also start to look better. The app is a fun and easy to use way to size up you and your friends and family. With dietary suggestions, exercise, acupressure, meditation, and herbal tea suggestions, you can begin to really personalize and monitor your wellness.

Funny thing you don't know about me?

Long bathroom lines are when I think 'civility' has gone too far and infrastructure building codes not far enough.

What is something quirky about you?

I'm as comfortable (and possibly more so) sleeping outside camping as I am in luxury hotels.

What's next?

I'm working on the next couple of books already. I've got one which is going to focus on the body map, looking at specific imbalances, diseases, and body parts and what they commonly point to as weaknesses in our mental/emotional/spiritual experience. I'm also working on one specifically related to overcoming chronic illness. I believe this whole idea of chronic illness when it pertains to internal dysfunction needs to be completely rethought. So much of our 'chronic illness' today is either preventable or persists because the treatments are terrible, diagnoses are unhelpful and actually inhibiting the process, and/or people aren't empowered enough to actually believe that they can feel better. The body turns on and off illness much more than we even realize. So much of chronic illness isn't about saying, "why am I sick all the time?" rather "why does my body continue to react to certain triggers time and time again?" If we can discover and defuse those triggers, our entire story gets rewritten.

This idea of overcoming chronic illness is something I am very passionate about. When we look at the cost of 'chronic illness' it is a burden that could cripple our healthcare industry. While a few pharmaceutical companies are making huge profits, quality of life is diminishing for everyone else. This can all change, and part of the change will come when we start asking the question, "Why do we assume that this particular illness is going to be ongoing and persistent?"

UNLEARNING
STRESS CREATING AN EASIER
HEALTHIER & MORE BALANCED LIFE

JAMES ROHR, L.Ac

Endnotes

1. Rakel, D 2007--Integrative medicine — *(Back to Read : Pg-5)*

2. This creates an overall net gain in the parasympathetic system, called 'respiratory sinus arrhythmia' -bmedreport.com/archives/8309. — *(Back to Read : Pg-5)*

3. http://www.soothingsoul.com/prod_daily_relaxer.htm — *(Back to Read : Pg-7)*

4. http://www.michellealva.com/ — *(Back to Read : Pg- 8)*

5. http://www.livestrong.com/article/370785-food-to-help-breathing/ — *(Back to Read : Pg-9)*

6. http://www.leastea.com/index.php?lang=ENGand-page=Page_T_10b — *(Back to Read : Pg-12)*

7. Willmann, Anna. "The Japanese Tea Ceremony". In Heilbrunn Timeline of Art History. New York: The Metropolitan Museum of Art, 2000–. http://www.metmuseum.org/toah/hd/jtea/hd_jtea.htm (April 2011) — *(Back to Read : Pg-12)*

8. http://www.asia-art.net/japanese_tea.html — *(Back to Read : Pg-13)*

9. http://issoantea.com/ — *(Back to Read : Pg-13)*

10. http://chriskresser.com/9-steps-to-perfect-health-6-manage-your-stress — *(Back to Read : Pg-19)*

11. Wu-men poem: http://enlightenyourday.com/2008/04/14/timeless-relaxing-zen-quotes-to-soothe-your-being/#.T62J0WA9Pm0 — *(Back to Read : Pg-25)*

12. John Kabat-Zinn http://www.youtube.com/watch?v=3nw-wKbM_vJcandfeature=player_embedded — *(Back to Read : Pg-27)*

13. Full Catstrophe Living p. 175 — *(Back to Read : Pg-29)*

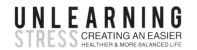

14. med/brain study: Eileen Luders, Florian Kurth, Emeran A. Mayer, Arthur W. Toga, Katherine L. Narr, Christian Gaser. The Unique Brain Anatomy of Meditation Practitioners: Alterations in Cortical Gyrification. Frontiers in Human Neuroscience, 2012; 6 DOI: 10.3389/fnhum.2012.0003 - University of California - Los Angeles (2012, March 14). Evidence builds that meditation strengthens the brain. ScienceDaily. Retrieved May 18, 2012, from http://www. sciencedaily.com/releases/2012/03/120314170647.htm — *(Back to Read : Pg-29)*

15. Lorenza S. Colzato, Ayca Ozturk, Bernhard Hommel. Meditate to Create: The Impact of Focused-Attention and Open-Monitoring Training on Convergent and Divergent Thinking. Frontiers in Psychology, 2012; 3 DOI: 10.3389/fpsyg.2012.00116 - Universiteit Leiden (2012, April 19). Meditation makes you more creative. ScienceDaily. Retrieved May 18, 2012, from http://www.sciencedaily.com/releases/2012/04/120419102317.htm — *(Back to Read : Pg-29)*

16. University of Pennsylvania (2007, June 25). Meditate To Concentrate. ScienceDaily. Retrieved May 18, 2012, from http://www.sciencedaily.com/releases/2007/06/070625193240.htm — *(Back to Read : Pg-29)*

17. Katherine MacLean, Clifford Saron, B. Alan Wallace et al. Intensive Meditation Training Improves Perceptual Discrimination and Sustained Attention. - Association for Psychological Science (2010, July 14). Meditation helps increase attention span. ScienceDaily. Retrieved May 18, 2012, from http://www. sciencedaily.com/releases/2010/07/100714121737.htm — *(Back to Read : Pg-29)*

18. American Academy of Sleep Medicine (2009, June 9). Meditation May Be An Effective Treatment For Insomnia. ScienceDaily. Retrieved May 18, 2012, from http://www.

sciencedaily.com/releases/2009/06/090609072719.htm
— *(Back to Read : Pg-29)*

19. University of Kentucky (2008, March 14). Meditation Can Lower Blood Pressure, Study Shows. ScienceDaily. Retrieved May 18, 2012, from http://www.sciencedaily.com/releases/2008/03/080314130430.htm — *(Back to Read : Pg-29)*

20. Medical College of Wisconsin (2009, November 16). Transcendental Meditation helped heart disease patients lower cardiac disease risks by 50 percent. ScienceDaily. Retrieved May 18, 2012, from http://www.sciencedaily.com/releases/2009/11/091116163204.htm — *(Back to Read : Pg-29)*

21. Christopher A. Brown, Anthony K.P. Jones. Meditation experience predicts less negative appraisal of pain: Electrophysiological evidence for the involvement of anticipatory neural responses. Pain, 2010; DOI: 10.1016/j.pain.2010.04.017 - University of Manchester (2010, June 2). Meditation reduces the emotional impact of pain, study finds. ScienceDaily. Retrieved May 18, 2012, from http://www.sciencedaily.com/releases/2010/06/100602091315.htm — *(Back to Read : Pg-29)*

22. Association for Psychological Science (2011, July 7). Teaching the neurons to meditate. ScienceDaily. Retrieved May 18, 2012, from http://www.sciencedaily.com/releases/2011/07/110707173321.htm — *(Back to Read : Pg-30)*

23. Jeffrey Thompson http://www.neuroacoustic.com/biotuning.html — *(Back to Read : Pg-36)*

24. Martin Jones, Feast, http://fds.oup.com/www.oup.com/pdf/13/9780199209019.pdf (23/36) — *(Back to Read : Pg-38)*

25. M. Hyman, Blood Sugar Solution, p. 85 — *(Back to Read : Pg-38)*

26. M. Hyman, The Blood Sugar Solution p.83. — *(Back to Read : Pg-39)*

27. "What are Humans Adapated For?" A lecture delivered by Daniel E. Lieberman, Professor of Human Evolutionary Biology, Harvard University http://www.fas.harvard.edu/~skeleton/danlhome.html for the Ancestral Health Symposium 2012. — *(Back to Read : Pg-39)*

28. Loren Cordain, Saturated Fat Consumption in Ancestral Human Diets: Implications for Contemporary Intakes. Chapter 8 in Phytochemicals: Nutrient-Gene Interactions edited by Mark S. Meskin, Wayne R. Bidlack and R. Keith Randolph, CRC Taylor and Francis Group p. 116. http://thepaleodiet.com/published-research/crc-chapter-2006a-3/ — *(Back to Read : Pg-39)*

29. chronic constipation statistic: http://digestive.niddk.nih.gov/statistics/statistics.aspx — *(Back to Read : Pg-40)*

30. Statistics on digestive disorders: http://scdlifestyle.com/2012/07/are-you-trapped-in-the-digestive-disease-epidemic/ — *(Back to Read : Pg-40)*

31. Crohn's Disease: http://www.ncbi.nlm.nih.gov/pubmedhealth/PMH0001295/ — *(Back to Read : Pg-40)*

32. Ulcerative colitis: http://www.ncbi.nlm.nih.gov/pubmedhealth/PMH0001296/ — *(Back to Read : Pg-40)*

33. Paul Jaminet, PhD: http://perfecthealthdiet.com/2010/07/ulcerative-colitis-a-devastating-gut-disease/ — *(Back to Read : Pg-40)*

34. Celiac disease: http://www.ncbi.nlm.nih.gov/pubmedhealth/PMH0001280/ — *(Back to Read : Pg-40)*

35. IBS: http://www.ncbi.nlm.nih.gov/pubmedhealth/PMH0001292/ — *(Back to Read : Pg-40)*

36. Hyman, UltraSimple Diet, p. 47 — *(Back to Read : Pg-42)*

37. Paul Jaminet, PhD. and Shou-Ching Shih Jaminet, Ph.D, Perfect Health Diet: Regain Health and Lose Weight by Eating the Way You Were Meant to Eat (Scribner) — *(Back to Read : Pg-42)*

38. Robb Wolf, http://robbwolf.com/what-is-the-paleo-diet/ — *(Back to Read : Pg-43)*

39. http://healthcoachpenny.com/vegetable-oil-is-people/ — *(Back to Read : Pg-45)*

40. Sally Fallon and Mary G. Enig, PhD, Lacto-Fermentation, January 2000: http://www.westonaprice.org/food-features/lacto-fermentation — *(Back to Read : Pg-46)*

41. http://blogs.discovermagazine.com/notrocketscience/2010/08/03/you-are-what-you-eat---how-your-diet-defines-you-in-trillions-of-ways/ — *(Back to Read : Pg-47)*

42. tips on how to incorporate more fermented stuff: http://www.cheeseslave.com/got-bacteria-10-reasons-to-eat-fermented-foods/ — *(Back to Read : Pg-47)*

43. Guyenet http://wholehealthsource.blogspot.com/2010/06/fermented-grain-recipes-from-around.html — *(Back to Read : Pg-47)*

44. Mother Earth News tested pastured eggs from around the US in 2007 and compared them to the listings in the USDA Nutrient Database – via http://wholehealthsource.blogspot.com/2009/05/pastured-eggs.html — *(Back to Read : Pg-49)*

45. Chris Masterjohn on nutrients in egg yolk: http://www.cholesterol-and-health.com/Egg_Yolk.html — *(Back to Read : Pg-49)*

46. Guyenet http://www.youtube.com/watch?v=HC20OoIgG_Y — *(Back to Read : Pg-50)*

47. http://news.sciencemag.org/sciencenow/2011/04/the-curse-of-the-mummies-arteries.html — *(Back to Read : Pg-51)*

48. http://www.uci.edu/features/2011/04/feature_mummy_110404.html — *(Back to Read : Pg-51)*

49. http://www.psychologytoday.com/blog/evolutionary-psychiatry/201108/wheat-and-serious-mental-illness — *(Back to Read : Pg-52)*

50. fast food and depression: Almudena Sánchez-Villegas, Estefania Toledo, Jokin de Irala, Miguel Ruiz-Canela, Jorge Pla-Vidal, Miguel A Martínez-González. Fast-food and commercial baked goods consumption and the risk of depression. Public Health Nutrition, 2011; 15 (03): 424 DOI: 10.1017/S1368980011001856 - June 6, 2012, from http://www.sciencedaily.com /releases/2012/03/120330081352.htm via Emily Deans, MD: http://evolutionarypsychiatry.blogspot.com/2012/04/fast-food-only-makes-us-happy-via-power_08.html — *(Back to Read : Pg-52)*

51. http://balancedbites.com/2011/04/the-dish-on-sugar-sweeteners.html — *(Back to Read : Pg-52)*

52. http://www.marksdailyapple.com/the-definitive-guide-to-sugar/#axzz25H0qfxGs — *(Back to Read : Pg-52)*

53. http://wholehealthsource.blogspot.com/2012/02/is-sugar-fattening.html — *(Back to Read : Pg-52)*

54. Julia Ross, Diet Cure, p.7. — *(Back to Read : Pg-52)*

55. Kessler, End of Overeating, p. 37. — *(Back to Read : Pg-53)*

56. Kessler, End of Overeating, p. 12. — *(Back to Read : Pg-53)*

57. http://www.wildfermentation.com/making-sauerkraut-2/#comment-194 — *(Back to Read : Pg-55)*

58. http://perfecthealthdiet.com/recommended-supplements/ — *(Back to Read : Pg-56)*

59. h t t p : / / w w w . s c i e n c e d a i l y . c o m / releases/2011/10/111020105904.htm — *(Back to Read : Pg-56)*

60. University of Zurich (2012, June 14). Training character strengths makes you happy. ScienceDaily. Retrieved September 14, 2012, from http://www.sciencedaily.com/ releases/2012/06/120614074940.htm — *(Back to Read : Pg-59)*

61. Kent State University (2008, November 27). Want To Be Happier? Be More Grateful. ScienceDaily. Retrieved September 14, 2012, from http://www.sciencedaily.com/ releases/2008/11/081125113005.htm — *(Back to Read : Pg-59)*

62. American Psychological Association (APA) (2012, August 5). Growing up grateful gives teens multiple mental health benefits. ScienceDaily. Retrieved September 14, 2012, from http:// www.sciencedaily.com/releases/2012/08/120806093938.htm — *(Back to Read : Pg-59)*

63. Adam Grant and Jane Dutton. Beneficiary or Benefactor: The Effects of Reflecting about Receiving versus Giving on Prosocial Behavior. Psychological Science, 2012. Association for Psychological Science (2012, August 10). Thinking about giving, not receiving, motivates people to help others. ScienceDaily. Retrieved September 14, 2012, from http:// www.sciencedaily.com/releases/2012/08/120810112812.htm — *(Back to Read : Pg-59)*

64. In Personal Relationships. Wiley-Blackwell (2010, May 24). It's the little things: Everyday gratitude as a booster shot for romantic relationships. ScienceDaily. Retrieved September 14, 2012, from http://www.sciencedaily.com/ releases/2010/05/100524072912.htm — *(Back to Read : Pg-59)*

65. Yeri Cho, Nathanael J. Fast. Power, defensive denigration, and the assuaging effect of gratitude expression. Journal of

Experimental Social Psychology, 2012; 48 (3): 778 DOI: 10.1016/j.jesp.2011.1. University of Southern California (2012, March 29). How to handle your insecure boss. ScienceDaily. Retrieved September 14, 2012, from http://www.sciencedaily.com /releases/2012/03/120329100901.htm — *(Back to Read : Pg-59)*

66. http://www.cchrint.org/tag/antianxiety/ — *(Back to Read : Pg-70)*

67. Craig A. Olsson, Rob McGee, Shyamala Nada-Raja, Sheila M. Williams. A 32-Year Longitudinal Study of Child and Adolescent Pathways to Well-Being in Adulthood. Journal of Happiness Studies, 2012; DOI: 10.1007/s10902-012-9369-8 - Springer Science+Business Media (2012, August 2). Early relationships, not brainpower, key to adult happiness. ScienceDaily. Retrieved September 16, 2012, from http://www.sciencedaily.com/releases/2012/08/120802092222.htm — *(Back to Read : Pg-71)*

68. Lianne M. Kurina, Kristen L. Knutson, Louise C. Hawkley, John T. Cacioppo, Diane S. Lauderdale, Carole Ober. Loneliness Is Associated with Sleep Fragmentation in a Communal Society. Sleep, 2011; DOI: 10.5665/sleep.1390 via American Academy of Sleep Medicine (2011, November 2). How lonely you are may impact how well you sleep, research shows. ScienceDaily. Retrieved September 16, 2012, from h h t t p : / / w w w . s c i e n c e d a i l y . c o m / releases/2011/11/111101095302.htm — *(Back to Read : Pg-71)*

69. Chris Segrin, Stacey Passalacqua. Functions of Loneliness, Social Support, Health Behaviors, and Stress in Association With Poor Health. Health Communication, 2010; 25 (4): 312 DOI: 10.1080/10410231003773334 via University of Arizona (2010, June 23). Loneliness, poor health appear to be linked. ScienceDaily. Retrieved September 16, 2012, from http://www.sciencedaily.com/releases/2010/06/100622091746.htm — *(Back to Read : Pg-71)*

70. The morning urine of lonely people was found to contain higher levels of the stress hormone, epinephrine, according to research by John Cacioppo, the director of the Center for Cognitive and Social Neuroscience at the University of Chicago and world's leading expert on loneliness. "When we drew blood from our older adults and analyzed their white cells," he continues, "we found that loneliness somehow penetrated the deepest recesses of the cell to alter the way genes were being expressed." http://www.theatlantic.com/magazine/archive/2012/05/is-facebook-making-us-lonely/308930/. — *(Back to Read : Pg-71)*

71. Cacioppo et al. What Are the Brain Mechanisms on Which Psychological Processes Are Based? Perspectives on Psychological Science, 2009; 4 (1): 10 DOI: 10.1111/j.1745-6924.2009.01094.x via University of Chicago (2009, February 17). Loneliness Affects How The Brain Operates. ScienceDaily. Retrieved September 16, 2012, from http://www.sciencedaily.com/releases/2009/02/090215151800.htm — *(Back to Read : Pg-71)*

72. "We detected an extraordinary pattern of contagion that leads people to be moved to the edge of the social network when they become lonely," explains University of Chicago researcher psychologist John Cacioppo, is a leading scholarly expert on loneliness. "The data showed that lonely people "infected" the people around them with loneliness, and those people moved to the edges of social circles." University of Chicago (2009, December 2). Loneliness can be contagious. ScienceDaily. Retrieved September 16, 2012, from http://www.sciencedaily.com/releases/2009/12/091201084047.htm — *(Back to Read : Pg-71)*

73. http://www.theatlantic.com/magazine/archive/2012/05/is-facebook-making-us-lonely/308930/ — *(Back to Read : Pg-71)*

74.   http://www.theatlantic.com/magazine/archive/2012/05/ is-facebook-making-us-lonely/308930/   — *(Back to Read : Pg-71)*

75.   http://www.theatlantic.com/magazine/archive/2012/05/ is-facebook-making-us-lonely/308930/   — *(Back to Read : Pg-71)*

76.   http://newsinhealth.nih.gov/2009/February/feature1.htm — *(Back to Read : Pg-73)*

77.   h t t p : / / w w w . t e l e g r a p h . c o . u k / n e w s / worldnews/1570492/A-dog-is-just-for-the-afternoon.html — *(Back to Read : Pg-73)*

78.   http://www.boston.com/news/local/breaking_news/2008/06/ ban_proposed_fo.html   — *(Back to Read : Pg-73)*

79.   European Society of Cardiology (ESC) (2011, August 28). Laughter has positive impact on vascular function. ScienceDaily. Retrieved April 1, 2012, from http://www.sciencedaily.com/ releases/2011/08/110828101806.htm   — *(Back to Read : Pg-74)*

80.   Centered   Silliness,   http://www.dailyom.com/ articles/2005/584.html. — *(Back to Read : Pg-74)*

81.   Mama Gena's School of Womanly Arts: Using the Power of Pleasure to Have Your Way with the World (2002) by Regina Thomashauer - http://www.mamagenas.com/books/ — *(Back to Read : Pg-76)*

82.   Kayser, M.; Brauer, S.; Weiss, G.; Underhill, P. A.; Roewer, L.; Schiefenhövel, W.; Stoneking, M. (2000). "Melanesian origin of Polynesian Y chromosomes". Current Biology 10 (20): 1237–1246.   doi:10.1016/S0960-9822(00)00734-X.   PMID 11069104   via   http://en.wikipedia.org/wiki/Polynesia — *(Back to Read : Pg-79)*

83.   The Qi that provides the basis for vitality and stamina imbued to you during conception and development as a fetus, your body's original Qi, is the Ancestral Qi. When you eat and

process food, part of its Qi goes to the lungs and another part to the heart, where it is turned into blood. The result of digestion and metabolism is Food Qi. The primary motive force for circulation is the Gathering Qi and as it is further refined and enters the last stage of transformation, it becomes True Qi. True Qi is what flows through the meridians and is impacted by an acupuncture needle, and has two interesting qualities: (1) It nourishes and fuels the internal organs as Nutritive Qi and as such is closely related the blood and is the primary Qi that is cultivated during our lifetime; and (2) it flows across the outer layers of the body, protecting us as Defensive Qi . Defensive Qi is similar in concept to the Western idea of an immune system and flows both on the outer layer of the skin and deeper, at the primary level of the acupuncture meridians. — *(Back to Read : Pg-81)*

84. http://www.mayoclinic.com/health/chemo-brain/DS01109 — *(Back to Read : Pg-82)*

85. http://www.macmillan.org.uk/Cancerinformation/ Livingwithandaftercancer/Physicalactivity/Physicalactivi- tyvideos.aspx - Macmillan Cancer Support via http://fitness. mercola.com/sites/fitness/archive/2012/09/21/ exercise-helps-cancer-patients.aspx?e_cid=20120921_DNL_ art_1#_edn4 — *(Back to Read : Pg-82)*

86. Cardiovascular Risk of High- Versus Moderate-Intensity Aerobic Exercise in Coronary Heart Disease Patients. Øivind Rognmo; Trine Moholdt; Hilde Bakken; Torstein Hole; Per Mølstad; Nils Erling Myhr; Jostein Grimsmo; Ulrik Wisløff. CIRCULATIONAHA.112.123117. Published online before print August 9, 2012, doi: 10.1161/ CIRCULATIO- NAHA.112.123117 — *(Back to Read : Pg-83)*

87. http://pennstatehershey.adam.com/content.aspx?produc- tId=16andgid=55927 — *(Back to Read : Pg-83)*

88. Congcong He, Michael C. Bassik, Viviana Moresi, Kai Sun, Yongjie Wei, Zhongju Zou, Zhenyi An, Joy Loh, Jill Fisher, Qihua Sun, Stanley Korsmeyer, Milton Packer, Herman I.

May, Joseph A. Hill, Herbert W. Virgin, Christopher Gilpin, Guanghua Xiao, Rhonda Bassel-Duby, Philipp E. Scherer, Beth Levine. Exercise-induced BCL2-regulated autophagy is required for muscle glucose homeostasis. Nature, 2012; DOI: 10.1038/nature10758 - UT Southwestern Medical Center (2012, January 22). Health benefits of exercise may depend on cellular degradation. ScienceDaily. Retrieved September 21, 2012, from http://www.sciencedaily.com/releases/2012/01/120120184528.htm — (Back to Read : Pg-83)

89. Lauren E. McCullough, Sybil M. Eng, Patrick T. Bradshaw, Rebecca J. Cleveland, Susan L. Teitelbaum, Alfred I. Neugut, Marilie D. Gammon. Fat or fit: The joint effects of physical activity, weight gain, and body size on breast cancer risk. Cancer, 2012; DOI: 10.1002/cncr.27433 - Wiley-Blackwell (2012, June 25). Exercise, even mild physical activity, may reduce breast cancer risk. ScienceDaily. Retrieved September 21, 2012, from http://www.sciencedaily.com/releases/2012/06/120625065334.htm — (Back to Read : Pg-83)

90. Eric B. Rimm. A Prospective Study of Weight Training and Risk of Type 2 Diabetes Mellitus in Men Weight Training and Risk of Type 2 Diabetes. Archives of Internal Medicine, 2012; : 1 DOI: 10.1001/archinternmed.2012.3138 - Harvard School of Public Health (2012, August 6). Weight training linked to reduced risk of type 2 diabetes. ScienceDaily. Retrieved September 21, 2012, from http://www.sciencedaily.com/releases/2012/08/120806161816.htm — (Back to Read : Pg-83)

91. A systematic review published in The Cochrane Library by a team from the Karolinska Institute in Stockholm, Sweden. Wiley-Blackwell (2011, October 4). Regular exercise improves health of people with long-term kidney disease, study suggests. ScienceDaily. Retrieved September 21, 2012, from http://www.sciencedaily.com/releases/2011/10/111004221112.htm — (Back to Read : Pg-83)

UNLEARNING STRESS CREATING AN EASIER HEALTHIER & MORE BALANCED LIFE

JAMES ROHR, L.Ac

92. F. Langlois, T. T. M. Vu, K. Chasse, G. Dupuis, M.-J. Kergoat, L. Bherer. Benefits of Physical Exercise Training on Cognition and Quality of Life in Frail Older Adults. The Journals of Gerontology Series B: Psychological Sciences and Social Sciences, 2012; DOI: 10.1093/geronb/gbs069 - University of Montreal (2012, September 6). Even the very elderly and frail can benefit from exercise. ScienceDaily. Retrieved September 21, 2012, from http://www.sciencedaily.com/releases/2012/09/120906182008.htm — *(Back to Read : Pg-83)*

93. Yu-Wen Chen, Yung-Tsung Li, Yu Chung Chen, Zong-Ying Li, Ching-Hsia Hung. Exercise Training Attenuates Neuropathic Pain and Cytokine Expression After Chronic Constriction Injury of Rat Sciatic Nerve. Anesthesia and Analgesia, 2012; 114 (6): 1330 DOI: 10.1213/ANE.0b013e31824c4ed4 - International Anesthesia Research Society (IARS) (2012, June 1). How Does Exercise Affect Nerve Pain?. ScienceDaily. Retrieved September 21, 2012, from http://www.sciencedaily.com/releases/2012/06/120601120513.htm — *(Back to Read : Pg-83)*

94. According to a study by kinesiology researchers in the University of Maryland School of Public Health published in the journal Medicine and Science in Sports and Exercise - University of Maryland (2012, September 13). Exercise may protect against future emotional stress, study shows. ScienceDaily. Retrieved September 21, 2012, from http://www.sciencedaily.com/releases/2012/09/120913123629.htm — *(Back to Read : Pg-83)*

95. Research abstract presented the 22nd Annual Meeting of the Associated Professional Sleep Societies (APSS) by Giselle S. Passos of Federal University of Sao Paulo in Brazil - American Academy of Sleep Medicine (2008, June 12). Moderate Exercise Can Improve Sleep Quality Of Insomnia Patients. ScienceDaily. Retrieved September 21, 2012, from http://www.sciencedaily.

com/releases/2008/06/080611071129.htm — *(Back to Read : Pg-83)*

96. Ashish Sharma, M.D., Vishal Madaan, M.D., and Frederick D. Petty, M.D., Ph.D.. Exercise for Mental Health, Prim Care Companion J Clin Psychiatry. 2006; 8(2): 106. http://www.ncbi.nlm.nih.gov/pmc/articles/PMC1470658/ — *(Back to Read : Pg-83)*

97. http://www.drweil.com/drw/u/QAA400537/Stumped-by-Oxidative-Stress.html — *(Back to Read : Pg-83)*

98. L. G. Koch, O. J. Kemi, N. Qi, S. X. Leng, P. Bijma, L. J. Gilligan, J. E. Wilkinson, H. Wisloff, M. A. Hoydal, N. Rolim, P. M. Abadir, I. Van Grevenhof, G. L. Smith, C. F. Burant, O. Ellingsen, S. L. Britton, U. Wisloff. Intrinsic Aerobic Capacity Sets a Divide for Aging and Longevity. Circulation Research, 2011; DOI: 10.1161/CIRCRESAHA.111.253807 - The Norwegian University of Science and Technology (NTNU) (2011, September 30). Intrinsic aerobic exercise capacity linked to longevity. ScienceDaily. Retrieved September 21, 2012, from http://www.sciencedaily.com/releases/2011/09/110930102806.htm — *(Back to Read : Pg-84)*

99. http://www.mayoclinic.com/health/fitness/HQ00171 — *(Back to Read : Pg-85)*

100. http://www.acsm.org/about-acsm/media-room/news-releases/2011/08/01/acsm-issues-new-recommendations-on-quantity-and-quality-of-exercise — *(Back to Read : Pg-85)*

101. http://www.naturalnews.com/023602_sitting_fat_muscles.html — *(Back to Read : Pg-86)*

102. As part of a series of studies presented at the Second International Congress on Physical Activity and Public Health in Amsterdam, Hamilton by researcher Theodore Zderic and his team at the University of Missouri-Columbia – based on research they published in Diabetes. University of Missouri-Columbia

(2007, November 20). Sitting May Increase Risk Of Disease. ScienceDaily. Retrieved September 22, 2012, from http://www.sciencedaily.com/releases/2007/11/071119130734.htm — *(Back to Read : Pg-87)*

103. PGDipNutMed., PGDipSportExMed., BSc., BPhEd — *(Back to Read : Pg-88)*

104. http://thatpaleoguy.com/2011/04/18/survival-of-the-fittest/ — *(Back to Read : Pg-88)*

105. http://www.menshealth.com/fitness/army-training-guide — *(Back to Read : Pg-88)*

106. BMJ-British Medical Journal (2008, August 20). Alexander Technique Offers Long-term Relief For Back Pain. ScienceDaily. Retrieved September 22, 2012, from http://www.sciencedaily.com/releases/2008/08/080819213029.htm — *(Back to Read : Pg-89)*

107. Helen E. Tilbrook et al. Yoga for Chronic Low Back Pain A Randomized Trial. Annals of Internal Medicine, 2011 - University of York (2011, October 31). Yoga aids chronic back pain sufferers, study suggests. ScienceDaily. Retrieved September 22, 2012, from http://www.sciencedaily.com/releases/2011/10/111031220257.htm — *(Back to Read : Pg-89)*

108. http://www.movementdialogues.com/home/the-feldenkrais-method — *(Back to Read : Pg-89)*

109. http://www.thereporter.com.au/story/2012/04/17/polynesian-fitness-rage-shakes-up-logan/ — *(Back to Read : Pg-90)*

110. via http://www.besthealthmag.ca/get-healthy/fitness/the-8-most-unusual-workouts? — *(Back to Read : Pg-90)*

111. via http://lifehacker.com/5879536/how-sitting-all-day-is-damaging-your-body-and-how-you-can-counteract-it — *(Back to Read : Pg-91)*

112. via http://walking.about.com/od/measure/tp/pedometer.htm
— *(Back to Read : Pg-91)*

113. He was a well-known turn of the century American politician and leading orator of the period. — *(Back to Read : Pg-93)*

114. Gaetano Milanesi, Le lettere di Michelangelo Buonarroti pubblicati coi ricordi ed i contratti artistici, Florence, 1875, 620-623: — *(Back to Read : Pg-93)*

115. The numbers of failed Edison lightbulb attempts seem to vary with the telling, from a low of maybe 700 times to a whopping 10,000 failures. — *(Back to Read : Pg-109)*

116. http://www.neatorama.com/2007/10/23/10-kick-ass-facts-about-bruce-lee/ — *(Back to Read : Pg-111)*

117. http://www.innerchangemag.com/mysteryschool.htm — *(Back to Read : Pg-113)*

118. http://consciouslifenews.com/gregg-braden-living-heart-beauty-compassion-healing-master-plan-video-plus-transcript/1125953/ — *(Back to Read : Pg-114)*

119. We intend no disrespect to any doctors reading and have utmost respect for your training and desire to heal. Our goal here is to try and to help your patients be better partners in your collaborative work of healing. — *(Back to Read : Pg-115)*

120. http://www.greggbraden.com/press-and-media/rewriting-the-reality-code — *(Back to Read : Pg-116)*

121. Tali Sharot, Optimism Bias, p. 56 — *(Back to Read : Pg-116)*

122. Qi gong, often referred to as the internal martial art, helps you feel energy inside and out and channel that for self-healing. Over the years, I've had many clients tell me they were diagnosed with potentially fatal or catastrophic illnesses and Qi Gong has helped them to cope or completely overcome their diagnosis. — *(Back to Read : Pg-117)*